BACON & BUTTER

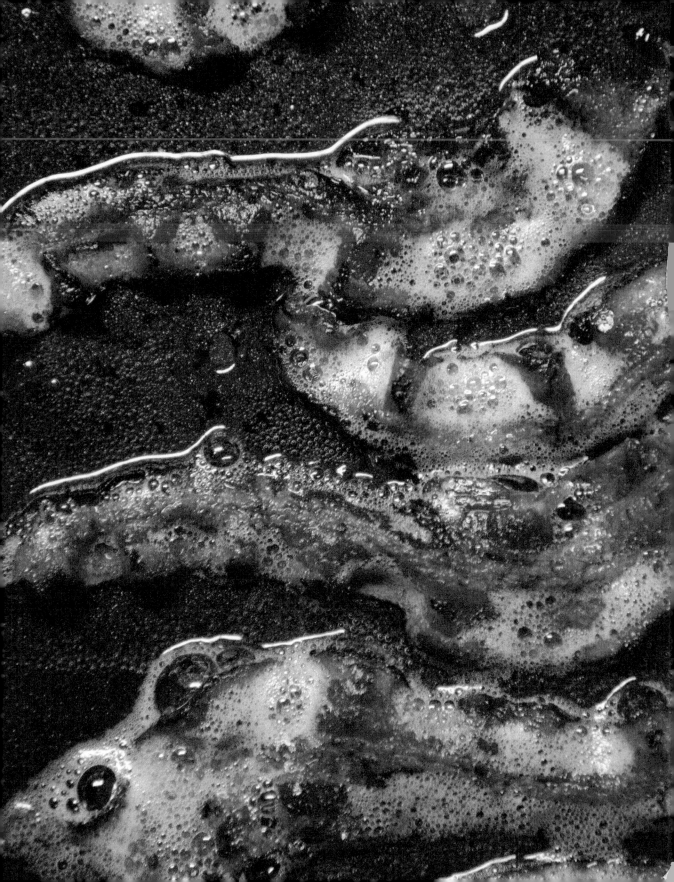

BACON & BUTTER

The Ultimate Ketogenic Diet Cookbook

BY CELBY RICHOUX

ROCKRIDGE
PRESS

QUICK START GUIDE

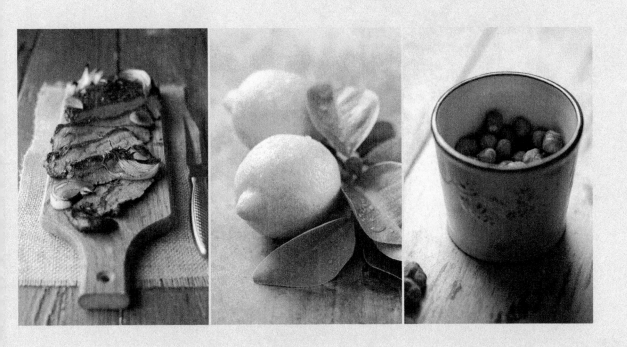

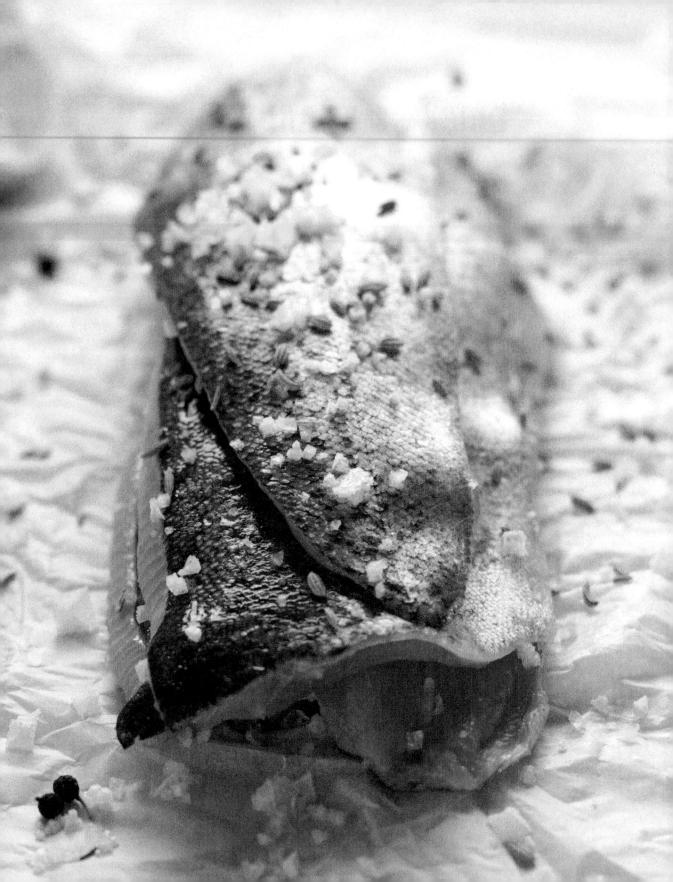

CONTENTS

MY STORY

When I began my journey with keto, I had slowly been gaining weight and suffering from headaches, gastrointestinal issues, mood swings, loss of concentration, and low energy levels for more than two years. I went through every diet fad or supplement there was, consulted multiple doctors to find out why I had these issues, and continued to gain weight despite following a "healthy diet." When my blood work came back as normal, they shrugged their shoulders and said, "Maybe you should eat more fruits and vegetables." Despite my experience, I knew another answer had to be out there. Eventually, I discovered keto.

> "I am finally able to control my weight and energy levels by eating the foods I love, and I have developed a new appreciation for my overall health and nutrition."

Like most dieters, I found the idea of using fat as a main fuel source for my body completely foreign. I had no idea what a macronutrient was or why one macronutrient may be better for me to utilize for energy than another. I believed that "good food" was anything with a low amount of fat or sugar, and "bad food" was everything else. It was very enlightening to go through my pantry and look at the carbohydrate content of some of my staple foods, like nutrition bars and whole-wheat products—I had been putting myself on an insulin-energy roller coaster without even realizing it. After a thorough overhaul of my carb-laden kitchen, I began the process of entering ketosis and embracing my new way of life.

During the first few weeks of keto, I had some incredibly positive changes in my mood, energy, and weight. Though it was hard to believe at first, as time went on and the symptoms I had suffered from faded, the proof was hard to ignore. I began to accept the fact that not only could my body operate on an alternative fuel source, but that source could also help my metabolism melt away pounds and cure ailments in a way I never thought possible.

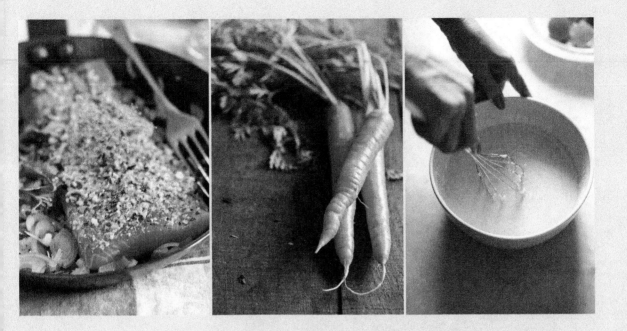

As I adapted to living in ketosis I wondered, "Why isn't everyone doing this?" I remembered from my research that people were using this diet, but many were doing so to control seizure disorders and other medical issues— not to lose weight. According to the Epilepsy Foundation, the keto diet allows many epileptics to live a much more controlled life—some are even completely free of symptoms—which is a miracle for those who once suffered dozens to hundreds of seizures per day. Even though I came to keto with different goals, with this kind of healing history the efficacy of the diet was undeniable. It very quickly shifted from being a "diet" to a "lifestyle" for me.

The impact that keto has had on my life is incredible. I am finally able to control my weight and energy levels by eating the foods I love, and I have developed a new appreciation for my overall health and nutrition. Recreating some of my favorite meals so they are keto-friendly—and discovering new ones—has been a big part of my success with the diet. Many of those recipes are included here in this book for you. I hope you enjoy them, and that your journey with keto is beneficial to your health and well-being, too.

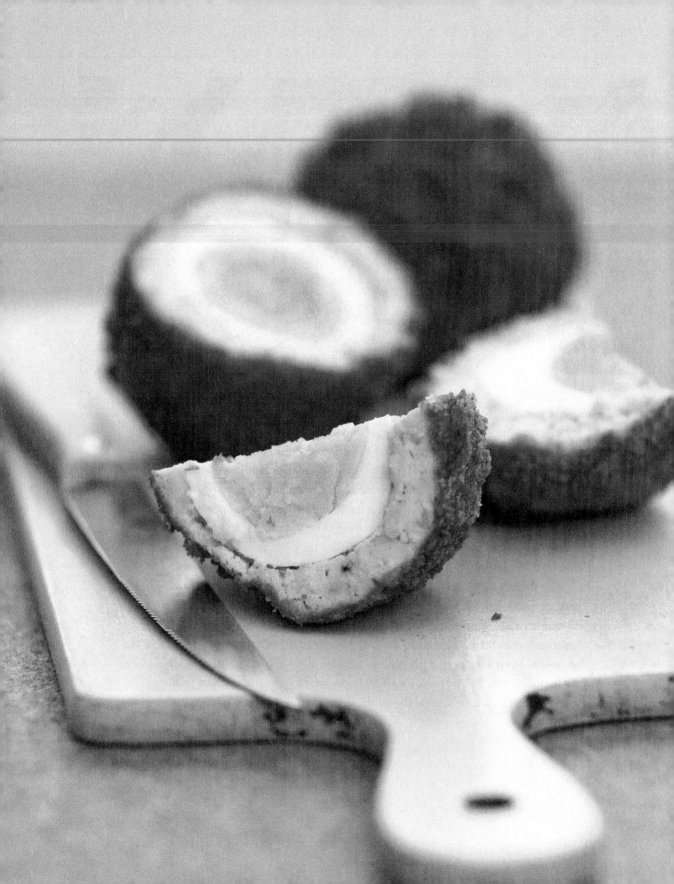

CHAPTER

1

OF RATIOS AND RATIONS

Bacon for breakfast, ham and cheese roll-ups for lunch, buttered asparagus and steak for dinner. You're not dreaming—this is a snapshot of a day in the life of a keto dieter.

The generally accepted claim that fat is not your friend is about to be thrown out the window. Say good-bye to the low-fat 100-calorie cookie snack packs and fat-free dairy creamer. When adopting a keto diet, fat is your best friend, and sugar-rich carbohydrates are your worst enemy. Though keto is called a diet, it is also a lifestyle change centered on seeking to better one's health through an understanding of the human body and basic nutrition.

In its simplest form, the keto diet is a **high-fat**, **moderate-protein**, **low- to no-carbohydrate diet** that encourages the body to stop burning carbohydrate and protein for fuel in favor of burning fat, thus entering a state called ketosis.

What Is Ketosis?

Ketosis is a metabolic state in which the body uses dietary and bodily fats as its primary energy source. Traditionally, the body operates in a state of glycolysis, deriving its energy from blood glucose. When in a state of ketosis, however, the body's energy instead comes from ketone bodies, produced when the body burns fat for fuel. The adoption of the ketogenic diet, then, forces the body to adapt to using ketones for energy through dietary deprivation of glucose/sugar, which causes glycogen stores to deplete. Once these stores deplete, the body switches to burning fats for fuel, and the trace amounts of glycogen required for brain function are acquired from stores in the liver.

A study in *Obesity Reviews* also shows that a keto diet is a proven way for dieters to lose weight safely and effectively. Used with proper understanding and research, a ketogenic diet is appropriate for almost anyone, as it helps promote cardiovascular health, stable cholesterol levels, and mental focus.

KETOSIS AND KETOACIDOSIS: THE DIFFERENCE

Ketosis and ketoacidosis, though similar in name, are extremely different metabolic states. **Ketosis**, as defined in this chapter, is a state in which the body "flips" from utilizing carbohydrate for energy to using fat. This happens through dietary deprivation of carbohydrate, which creates a regulated and controlled amount of ketones in the body.

Ketoacidosis, on the other hand, is a dangerous metabolic state brought on by a lack of insulin in the body and the presence of massive quantities of ketones. This state is usually seen in type 1 diabetics, and it should be monitored closely by anyone suffering from the disease.

Macronutrients

Macronutrients fuel the body. There are three "macros": *fat, protein,* and *carbohydrate.* The macronutrient makeup of a keto diet is:

- 60 to 80 percent *fat*
- 20 to 35 percent *protein*
- 0 to 5 percent *carbohydrate*

All foods have macronutrient content, even though some may seem to contain only carbs. Kale for example, is mostly carbohydrate, but also contains a healthy portion of protein. All macronutrients are considered integral, but the human body is capable of obtaining its energy primarily from protein and fat. And, while carbohydrate is an essential nutrient for function, the trace amount of carbohydrates needed for the body can be acquired from vegetables instead of grains. This distinction, together with the focus on getting the majority of your caloric intake from fat, is the nutritional basis of the ketogenic diet.

Keto is different from other low-carb diets because the goal is not only to restrict carbohydrate intake, but also to enter and maintain a state of ketosis. Many diets tout "low carb" as one of the cornerstones of success, but most do not require as stringent a restriction of carbohydrates in overall caloric intake as the keto diet does. Sticking to the macronutrient percentages is integral to keeping the body in a state of ketosis. A study from the *European Journal of Clinical Nutrition* found that when in ketosis, our bodies function more smoothly, no longer experiencing energy highs and lows triggered by the insulin response from a carbohydrate-based diet. Being in ketosis also helps maintain concentration, as our bodies are not constantly struggling for fuel stability and can focus on the task at hand.

Try this keto calculator to help determine the proper macronutrient breakdown for your body and lifestyle. The most common macronutrient breakdown for keto dieters is 65/30/5 (fat/protein/carbohydrate), but that varies depending on your level of activity and whether your goal is to lose weight. Find out what works best for you with this helpful calculator: keto-calculator.ankerl.com.

4:1 and 3:1 Ratios

When reading the recipes in this book, you will find the 4:1 or 3:1 distinction with the nutritional information. These ratios come from the classic ketogenic diet, developed for use by those with seizure disorders or other medical issues. Each of these ratios relates to the dietary units of fat in the recipe being four, or three, times the dietary units of the combined protein and carbohydrate content.

Because fat is energy-dense, with 9 kilocalories per gram (kcal/g) compared to 4 kcal/g for protein or carbohydrate, meals tend to be smaller and more filling when a 4:1 or 3:1 ratio is used. While perfect ratios are ideal, a recipe usually will fall closer to one of these ratios or the other rather than being exact.

WEIGHING AND LOGGING

Depending on your reason for adopting the keto diet, weighing and measuring food may be required. While eating a keto diet does allow your body to adapt to a fat-burning metabolic state, it does not mean that calories do not matter. If using the diet for weight loss, weighing your food for portion control early on is a good choice. This ensures that you know your true daily caloric intake. After adapting to the keto diet, you may find you can "eyeball" your portions without pulling out the scale.

In addition to weighing your food, a food log can also be helpful—not only for tracking calories, but also for determining which foods affect you in certain ways. For example, one day you might enjoy a large portion of spaghetti squash but find that it didn't agree with you. It is important to note which foods work for your body and which do not.

Net Carbohydrates

Since keto is a carbohydrate-restrictive diet, limiting your carbohydrate intake is key. When calculating your carbs for the day, it's important that you take into account the fiber content of whatever you have eaten. Even though fiber is a carbohydrate, it does not digest into glucose but instead passes through the body. *To render the net carbs of your food or recipe, always subtract the amount of fiber from the total carbohydrate amount.*

For example, looking at that side of broccoli you'll eat with dinner:

- 100g of broccoli contains 7g total carbohydrate and 3g of fiber.
- When we subtract the fiber (3g) from the total carbohydrates (7g) the net carbs in 100g of broccoli is 4g.

Most, if not all, of your carbohydrate intake should come from fibrous vegetables or low-glycemic fruit. A food is considered low-glycemic when it is low on the glycemic index. The glycemic index categorizes which foods have the most (high-glycemic) and least (low-glycemic) impact on blood sugar and insulin. Since one benefit of keto is a stable insulin response, high-glycemic fruits and vegetables should be avoided. An app like Low GI Diet Tracker will help you stay away from high-glycemic foods.

To shift the body into a state of ketosis, you must keep your daily net carbohydrate intake at or below 20 grams. This process takes between two to three weeks for the average person to achieve. Some bodies can maintain ketosis while taking in as much as 50 grams net carbohydrate per day. However, a daily intake of 20 grams net carbohydrate or lower is recommended to induce ketosis, and this level should be maintained for at least a few months until the body is fully keto-adapted. Once you know how individual foods affect you, experimenting with a higher threshold for daily carbohydrates is okay.

Low-Carb Foods to Enjoy

One of the best parts of the keto diet is the food. If you'd like a breakfast of bacon and eggs every day, you've got it. Have a craving for cream cheese? Try an onion chive dip with some celery sticks. The beauty of this diet is not only in its simplicity, but also in the ability to enjoy whole, nutritious foods that taste great. Most packaged foods are carbohydrate-based to improve shelf life. Your focus when grocery shopping should be on whole foods. This will reduce the risk of encountering hidden carbohydrates used as stabilizers in foods that may look keto-friendly, but are not. Following is an extensive list of food that is appropriate for the keto diet.

MEAT

Beef, all cuts	Lamb
Chicken, all cuts	Offal (organ meat)
Cured meats	Pork, all cuts
Duck	Quail
Eggs, all varieties	Veal
Goose	Venison

NUTS & SEEDS

Almonds	Peanuts
Brazil nuts	Pecans
Cashews	Pistachios
Chia seeds	Pumpkin seeds
Flaxseeds	Safflower seeds
Hazelnuts	Sesame seeds
Hemp seeds	Sunflower seeds
Macadamias	Walnuts

SEAFOOD

Bass	Oysters
Caviar	Salmon
Clams	Sardines
Crab	Scallops
Flounder	Shrimp
Halibut	Squid
Herring	Sole
Lobster	Tilapia
Mackerel	Trout
Mussels	Tuna, fresh and canned
Octopus	

LOW GLYCEMIC FRUITS & VEGETABLES

Arugula	Celery	Green beans	Rhubarb
Asparagus	Chicory greens	Jalapeño pepper	Spinach
Avocado	Cilantro	Lemon	Sprouts, alfalfa and other small seeds
Blackberries	Cranberries	Lettuce	Soybean
Bok choy	Cucumber	Lime	Swiss chard
Broccoli	Eggplant	Olives, green	Tomato
Broccoli raab	Endive	Parsley	Zucchini
Cabbage	Fennel	Radish	
Cauliflower	Garlic	Raspberries	

MODERATE GLYCEMIC FRUITS & VEGETABLES

Apple	Celeriac	Onion	Turnip
Artichoke	Kale	Pumpkin	Watermelon
Bell pepper	Kohlrabi	Snow peas	
Brussels sprouts	Mushrooms	Spaghetti squash	
Carrots, raw	Okra	Strawberries	

FATS & OILS

Almond butter	Macadamia oil
Almond oil	Olive oil
Avocado oil	Peanut butter, sugar-free
Butter	
Canola oil, in moderation	Peanut oil
	Safflower oil
Cocoa butter	Sesame oil
Coconut oil or MCT	Soybean oil
	Sunflower butter
Fish oil, cod liver	Sunflower oil
Flaxseed oil	Vegetable oil, in moderation
Grape seed oil	
Hemp seed oil	Walnut oil
Lard	

DAIRY

Almond milk, unsweetened	Greek yogurt, whole milk
Cheese, whole-milk varieties	Heavy cream
	Sour cream
Coconut cream	Soy milk, unsweetened
Coconut milk, unsweetened	
Cream cheese	Whipped cream, unsweetened

High-Carb Foods to Avoid

Reducing carbohydrate intake is the cornerstone of inducing ketosis. Avoid any high-carbohydrate foods completely to be successful with the keto diet. When we eat foods high in carbs, our bodies react by releasing insulin into the bloodstream to manage the increase in blood sugar created as those carbohydrates digest into sugar (glucose). If the glucose is not used productively for exercise, insulin forces the body to store it as fuel for later, which, in turn, becomes fat. A controlled trial by William S. Yancy Jr., Duke University School of Medicine, found that maintaining a stable insulin response through the carb-restricting keto diet not only allows your body to operate without those midday energy crashes, but it also encourages the release of fat stores acquired over years of constant insulin spikes.

Grains and Legumes

Unfortunately for the bread lovers out there, it does not matter if it's whole wheat, organic, *and* sprouted—it still translates into sugar once it enters your body. This grain and legume category includes pasta, baked goods, rice, beans, chips, crackers, pizza crust, and cereal. *All grains, grain-based foods, and legumes* (except peanuts) should be avoided while adapting to keto due to their high-carbohydrate content.

Everything bagels are one of my greatest weaknesses. Unfortunately, bagels happen to be one of the highest rated items on the glycemic index; sucrose has a glycemic index of 60, while the glycemic index of bagels averages 70. Needless to say, that love affair had to come to an end with the adoption of my keto lifestyle, but I still indulge in the smell anytime I pass by a bakery.

Dairy

While dairy is a staple food for the keto diet, some dairy foods are laden with carbohydrates. All milks (except those listed in the approved foods section) should be avoided, along with low-fat yogurt and cheese products. When shopping for dairy, look for grass-fed, full-fat options, which offer the most flavor and nutrients. If you have trouble finding them at your local grocery store, consider visiting a specialty store or nearby farmers' market.

Most Fruits and Certain Vegetables

Many favorite fruits sit high atop the glycemic index, and therefore, they are *not* allowed on the keto diet. Fruit may seem like an obvious healthy option when changing to a new diet, but most fruits cause a spike in insulin, which will knock you out of ketosis.

Fibrous vegetables are at the core of keto, and most vegetables with a high-fiber content can still be enjoyed. Outside of that, many staple vegetables lack fiber and also have high net carbohydrates. Vegetables like potatoes, corn, beets, peas, and winter squashes should be avoided.

Sugar

This seems obvious, but anything made with sugar is not allowed. Since keto depends on a low-insulin response from our bodies after we've eaten, anything with sugar will increase insulin thereby drastically reducing the efficacy and benefits of the diet.

Low-Fat Foods

Briefly mentioned previously in the dairy section, low-fat foods are not conducive to the keto diet since they lack the very foundation of it: fat. Another macronutrient (protein or carbohydrate) is usually substituted in low-fat foods so the product remains palatable, and that substitute usually consists of carbohydrates.

Special Mention: Spices, Sauces, and Condiments

With all of the meat and vegetables mentioned so far, you may be wondering how you're going to add some flavor to your meals. Fortunately, keto is not very restrictive when it comes to the flavor department. While there are a few instances in which certain spices, sauces, or condiments cannot be used, there is often a great substitute or a way for you to make your own—sans sugar or carbs. Over time, experimentation will yield some interesting flavor profiles you may not have known before.

"COUNTER" CULTURE

Keeping track of what you eat while on the ketogenic diet is extremely important. Without an accurate record, it can become difficult to maintain your macronutrients and stick to keto-approved foods. Watch your progress and log your foods daily with one of these online tools:

- MyFitnessPal (most popular)
- Lose It!
- CRON-O-Meter
- FatSecret

Sometimes, you may not be sure of a food's nutritional content. When in doubt, look up the nutritional information on one of these websites or apps:

- MyFitnessPal
- Fooducate
- SELFNutritionData
- CalorieKing
- CalorieCount

If you are worried you'll never enjoy a taco or pizza crust ever again, fear not—many low-carb bakeries exist and take orders online. Visit some of these online companies and distributors for low-carb tortillas and baking mixes, keto-friendly sauces, and more:

- Netrition
- Great Low Carb Bread Company
- Linda's Diet Delites
- Vitacost
- Low Carb Connoisseur

Spices

Spices will be your secret weapons as you navigate the keto diet. Most are very low in carbohydrates and rich in flavor. Loose, dry spices and fresh herbs are welcome and encouraged, but scrutinize prepackaged spice rubs, flavorings, and dried marinades carefully before using. Many prepackaged spice mixes contain sugar or other carbohydrate thickening and bonding agents, which should be avoided. Some spices also contain noticeable levels of net carbohydrates when used in larger portions. For most recipes, the amount required is negligible and usually too small to affect blood glucose levels. The *net carbohydrate* information for major spices *per tablespoon* follows.

- Allspice, ground, 3g
- Basil, dried, 0.9g
- Black pepper, 2.4g
- Cayenne pepper, 1.6g
- Cinnamon, 1.7g
- Cloves, 1.7g
- Cumin, ground, 2.1g
- Curry powder, 1.6g
- Garlic powder, 5.3g
- Ginger, ground, 3.1g
- Nutmeg, 2g
- Onion powder, 5.2g
- Oregano, ground, 0.4g
- Paprika, 1.2g
- Parsley, dried, 0.3g
- Pumpkin pie spice, 3.1g
- Sage, ground, 0.4g
- Tarragon, ground, 2g
- Thyme, ground, 1.1g
- Vanilla extract, imitation, 0.3g
- Vanilla extract, pure, 1.6g
- White pepper, 3g

Sauces

Sauces are havens for hidden sugars, so be sure to check the label before dousing a zucchini pasta dish with marinara or ribs with barbecue sauce. The degree to which certain sauces are sugared varies—tomato sauce, for example, can have as much as 10 grams of sugar per serving or just 1 gram of sugar per serving, depending on the manufacturer. Another thing to watch for is the use of thickeners. Usually carbohydrate-based, thickeners can turn an innocuous sauce like Alfredo into a high-carb one. Thickening agents such as agar agar, gelatin, nut and seed flours, or xanthan gum can help give keto sauces the consistency usually achieved with sugar. Following is a list of keto-friendly sauces.

- Alfredo sauce, thickener-free
- Barbecue sauce, sugar-free
- Béarnaise
- Buffalo sauce
- Cheese sauce
- Chimichurri
- Cream sauce
- Curry
- Hollandaise sauce
- Horseradish sauce
- Pasta sauce, sugar-free
- Pesto
- Pizza sauce, sugar-free

Condiments

Much like sauces, condiments that are usually considered savory might secretly pack a sugary punch, too. Ketchup is a front-runner in this department, as well as many marinades and salad dressings. If you are unable to find a sugar-free version of a favorite condiment, making it from scratch is an option. Salad dressing, for example, can be made very easily without the addition of sugar. A combination of mustard, vinegar, and oil will produce a light and refreshing dressing that can be adapted with herbs and spices in a variety of ways. Some popular keto-friendly condiments follow here:

- Capers
- Dill pickle relish
- Garlic chili paste
- Hot sauce
- Ketchup, sugar-free
- Mayonnaise
- Mustard, unsweetened
- Salad dressing, sugar-free
- Salsa, most varieties
- Soy sauce
- Vinegar, most clear or cider varieties
- Worcestershire sauce, sugar-free

Hydration and You

Hydration is an extremely important aspect of the keto diet, even more so than in a standard American diet. When your body enters ketosis, there is a diuretic effect in which more sodium and ketones are excreted through your urine than usual. In order to maintain healthy levels of hydration and electrolytes, make sure to add salt to your dishes or take a supplement (such as by adding an electrolyte drink mix to your drinking water). The recommendation for an average person's daily water intake is eight (8-ounce) glasses, or half a gallon.

Tips For Staying Hydrated

Since staying hydrated is crucial to your success on keto, you may sometimes have to trick yourself into remembering to drink water consistently. Some suggestions to improve your water intake are:

- Carry a large, refillable water bottle with you.
- Eat foods that contain significant amounts of water, like cucumber or celery.
- Replace your usual breakfast with a smoothie a few times a week.
- Drink a glass of water before bed, refill it, and leave it beside your bed to drink in the morning.
- Note that drinks like coffee and tea also count, as their diuretic effect is too weak to cause dehydration.

Cravings: Decoded

Cravings: We all get them, and so often, we succumb to them. What many people do not consider, though, is why they have cravings in the first place. Cravings tend to flare up when your body is lacking in certain nutrients. Fighting off cravings while on the keto diet is imperative since a single day of high-carbohydrate intake can bump you out of ketosis. If you find yourself craving something not allowed on the keto diet, try some of these suggested foods to help alleviate the urge to raid the nearest candy store.

Sweets

When craving sweets, your body may be trying to tell you it is missing some of its key nutrients. A deficiency in chromium, carbon, phosphorus, sulfur, or tryptophan will make you irritable and more likely to reach for a candy bar instead of a keto-friendly treat. To combat a craving for sweets, eat more dark, leafy vegetables; dairy; nuts; liver; chicken; and beef—all of which are all high in magnesium and the aforementioned key nutrients.

A special mention about chocolate cravings: You may need to add more foods high in magnesium to your diet. Raw nuts and seeds are great sources of magnesium. Unsweetened or high-percentage chocolate, like 90 percent to 100 percent cacao, can also be eaten in moderation.

Bread, Baked Goods, Pasta, and Rice

Considering how big a part grains play in the average American diet, a craving from this category will most likely occur sooner rather than later. This craving, likely fueled by a lack of nitrogen, can be put into check by eating more protein like fish, meat, and nuts.

Soda

While diet soda is allowed on keto if it does not affect your blood sugar, most dieters like to cut soda from their lives completely. If a craving does occur for your favorite can of pop, you could be low in calcium. Try reaching for some string cheese or a healthy serving of broccoli, kale, or other dark-green vegetable high in calcium at your next meal.

General Hunger

Oftentimes we are hungry seemingly for no reason. If drinking a large glass of water does not sate your hunger, you may be missing some key nutrients such as silicon, tryptophan, and tyrosine. Replenish your stores with nuts, seeds, cheese, spinach, liver, lamb, or vitamin C supplements.

Prior to keto, I was constantly hungry. It was almost maddening eating a hearty soup and sandwich for lunch and being hungry again at 2 PM. Luckily on the keto diet these bouts of "random" hunger are nearly eliminated. Sometimes you may even go without a pang of hunger for long periods of time; this is not abnormal, and becomes more common as you continue to adapt to the diet. If lunchtime rolls around and you're not hungry, don't look for reasons to eat; your body is capable of letting you know when you need fuel, especially while in ketosis.

Social Pressure

As can be expected in a world that eats mostly a high-carbohydrate diet, some family, friends, or coworkers may ask why you're eating so much fat.

FAT: NOT THE ENEMY

While keto may seem like a strange diet to some, there is a large amount of scientific evidence supporting its efficacy. In the References and Resources sections, you will find a variety of scientific studies, books, and websites dedicated to the most up-to-date research on the keto diet. Use these for further research or to share with family and friends.

Though you may be enthusiastic about keto, it's important to remember not everyone shares this enthusiasm or wants to eat this way. Much like politics and religion, food choices are a hot topic in debate. Many will take offense when the way they eat is called into question, even inadvertently; this was a lesson I learned early on, and it's something I stress to anyone I talk to who takes on the keto diet. No matter the situation or person—and whatever their reaction may be—know that this diet is for you and no one else. Above all, stay positive.

Family

Your family will likely be the people who are most vocal about, and interested in, your decision to adopt new eating habits. Whether they react with concern or encouragement, it's important to acknowledge their reaction. Explain that you have thoroughly researched the diet, and that you believe in its efficacy. My family was extremely supportive, but I also grew up in a household where the terms "fat-free" and "low-fat" were never uttered and no meal started without first passing around the butter.

Whatever your family's response, remind them that a supportive environment is the best one for anyone embarking on a new chapter in life. Some of your family members may even join you, in which case you may exceed weight loss or health goals and grow through the experience together.

Friends and Coworkers

Friends are the family you get to choose, and your coworkers are typically the people with whom you spend the most time. As such, these may be the first people that notice your change in symptoms or weight. While some offices thrive from group-related challenges, unless you are very close to your coworkers and some band together to join you, it's not recommended you spread the goodness of keto around your office. Some people may love the idea of a low-carb diet but they might struggle with adapting to the major metabolic change. For those that struggle, failing at keto while watching others succeed may deter them from trying a lifestyle change in the future. If someone asks in earnest to join you on your journey, you alone will know whether or not it is an ideal situation.

During my early success with the keto diet I had a coworker ask for information and guidance on how to join me. Excited to have an office buddy on the same journey, I obliged. Over the next few weeks I encouraged her as she brought in keto-friendly lunches and leftovers from the night before. Then, three weeks in, she gave up; discouraged by the difficulty of missing her favorite foods, it just wasn't for her. This was my first learning experience that keto isn't for everyone, but I'm still really glad she was open to trying it out.

As for close friends, inform them of your decision and let them know in advance that you would appreciate their support. Social gatherings tend to be the most likely times when I hear opposing views about my diet. I was at a party once when, in the heat of a moment, a friend pressed me to eat a sugar-laden cupcake, exclaiming, "How could a cupcake be worse for you than bacon?" You may be tempted to try to explain the complexities of keto and why it works, but I've learned that it's usually better to refrain from doing so unless specifically asked. While it may take time for friends to adjust to your new lifestyle, simply asking them to see that you are firm in your decision usually deters this behavior from happening repeatedly.

Food-Related Activities

Food is the focus of many of our daily activities and gatherings, and being prepared for such events will help you stay successful with the keto diet. If you plan to eat out with family, friends, or coworkers, try to look at the menu beforehand. This allows you to prepare your order and any questions you have in advance. When looking at the menu, look for dishes that are grilled or baked without sauce (unless an item is on the approved list), salads with dressing on the side, and sides made with leafy vegetables. My personal go-to restaurant meals are burgers without the bun, grilled meats with a side of buttered broccoli, buffalo chicken wings with bleu cheese and celery, and salads with keto-friendly add-ons.

Another situation you may encounter is an invitation to someone's home for dinner. Again, it's important to be prepared beforehand. Reach out to your host, if you're comfortable, to discuss your dietary needs. Oftentimes you can ask to bring your own meal portion if the meal being prepared is carbohydrate-based. If you encounter a situation with no obvious options or prior notice, try to work around the carbs and enjoy the non-carbohydrate portions of the meal. There was a day when my boss ordered pizza as a surprise, not realizing I couldn't partake. I simply ate the cheese and toppings, which was a tasty way to get my pizza fix without the carbs. While it may look strange sometimes, getting creative with what's available will carry you over until your next keto meal.

Making preparations and conscious decisions for any meal outside your home is key for the keto diet. Don't be afraid to speak up or say no if you're put in a situation where appropriate food is not available.

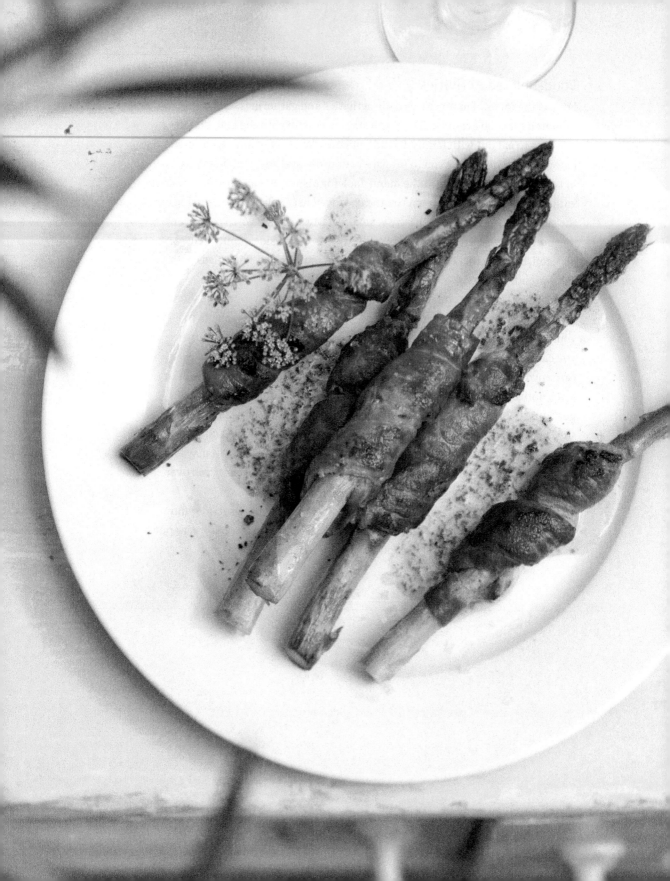

CHAPTER
2

BACON & BEYOND BREAKFAST

BUTTERED COFFEE

SERVES 1

TOTAL TIME: 15 MINUTES

Adding butter and oil to your coffee may seem a little far-fetched at first, but this recipe—blended so the oils combine with the coffee—delivers a smooth, delicious taste. It's sure to be your new favorite way to start the day. Since this recipe relies on so few ingredients, using high-quality butter is of the utmost importance for the final result. If you do not use medium-chain triglyceride (MCT) oil, you can substitute coconut oil.

1½ cups hot coffee

2 tablespoons unsalted butter

1½ tablespoons MCT oil, or coconut oil

Sugar-free sweetener

PER SERVING
(1 RECIPE)

RATIO: 4:1

CALORIES: 383

TOTAL FAT: 43.5g

CARBS: 0g

NET CARBS: 0g

FIBER: 0g

PROTEIN: 0.6g

1. Brew fresh coffee using your preferred method.

2. In a blender, add the coffee, butter, and oil. Blend until frothy, about 1 minute.

3. Flavor with a sweetener of your choice and enjoy.

INGREDIENT TIP: For this recipe, butter that comes from grass-fed cows should be used.

YOGURT PARFAIT WITH CHIA SEEDS

SERVES 1

TOTAL TIME: 20 MINUTES

If you are a yogurt lover, fear not: Yogurt is a treat that can be had on keto every once in a while, but only in its full-fat form. Creamy yogurt pairs well with the crunch of chia seeds and sliced almonds in this parfait recipe. Add fresh berries or a dash of cocoa powder for a real sweet treat.

1 cup full-fat yogurt

¼ cup unsweetened almond milk

2 tablespoons chia seeds

6 teaspoons sliced almonds, divided

¼ teaspoon cinnamon, divided

1. In a medium bowl, mix together the yogurt, almond milk, and chia seeds.
2. Pour one-third of the yogurt mixture into a tall glass. Sprinkle 2 teaspoons of almonds and a dash of cinnamon on top. Repeat two more times with the remaining yogurt, 4 teaspoons of almonds, and cinnamon, forming three layers.
3. Refrigerate to thicken for 5 to 10 minutes.

BACON & BEYOND BREAKFAST

PER SERVING
(1 RECIPE)

RATIO: 3:1

CALORIES: 434

TOTAL FAT: 33.4g

CARBS: 18.7g

NET CARBS: 6.7g

FIBER: 12g

PROTEIN: 14.4g

BAKED EGGS IN HAM CUPS

SERVES 2

PREP TIME: 5 MINUTES · COOK TIME: 15 MINUTES · TOTAL TIME: 20 MINUTES

If you're having company, these quick but satisfying breakfast cups are sure to please and will be fast on cleanup. They also serve as a great weekday breakfast— just pop the pan in the oven and grab one before you head out the door. Add a dash of hot sauce for a nice kick.

Cooking spray for cupcake pan

4 slices Black Forest ham

4 eggs

1 teaspoon dried parsley

1. Preheat the oven to 400°F.
2. Spray the cupcake pan.
3. Tuck one slice of ham into each cup. The ham will hang over the sides.
4. Crack one egg into each cup and garnish with the parsley.
5. Place the cupcake pan in the preheated oven. Cook for about 15 minutes, until the egg whites are cooked but the yolk is still runny.

PER SERVING
(2 EGGS WITH 2 SLICES HAM)

RATIO: 3:1

CALORIES: 221

TOTAL FAT: 13.9g

CARBS: 2.9g

NET CARBS: 2.1g

FIBER: 0.8g

PROTEIN: 20.5g

BACON, EGG, AND CHEESE CUPS

SERVES 4

PREP TIME: 5 MINUTES ❊ COOK TIME: 35 MINUTES ❊ TOTAL TIME: 40 MINUTES

A simple egg scramble inside a bacon cup is topped with cheese in this savory, compact meal made in a cupcake pan. I enjoy using this basic recipe and adding different cheeses or toppings, like mozzarella and basil or onion and Cheddar. Feel free to experiment to find your favorite way to enjoy these sunny breakfast cups.

6 bacon slices, divided

4 eggs, beaten

½ cup heavy (whipping) cream

¼ teaspoon salt

⅛ teaspoon freshly ground black pepper

½ cup shredded Monterey Jack cheese, divided

1. Preheat the oven to 350°F.

2. Wrap one bacon slice inside a cupcake tin around the edges, so it covers the sides of the tin. Repeat with three more slices in three more tins.

3. Cut the remaining two bacon slices into 2-inch pieces. Place 2 to 3 bacon pieces at the bottom of each bacon-wrapped cupcake tin so each is fully covered.

4. In a medium bowl, whisk together the eggs, heavy cream, salt, and pepper.

5. Pour the egg mixture evenly into the bacon-wrapped tins. Cover each with 2 tablespoons of cheese.

6. Carefully place the cupcake pan in the oven to avoid spillage. Bake for 35 minutes or until golden brown.

COOKING TIP: Save time using precooked bacon instead of uncooked bacon slices. Look for thick-cut precooked bacon since the regular cut tends to be very thin.

BACON & BEYOND BREAKFAST

PER SERVING
(1 EGG CUP)
RATIO: 3:1
CALORIES: 359
TOTAL FAT: 29g
CARBS: 1.5g
NET CARBS: 1.5g
FIBER: 0g
PROTEIN: 22.5g

CRUSTLESS QUICHE LORRAINE

SERVES 8

PREP TIME: 20 MINUTES ■ COOK TIME: 25 MINUTES ■ TOTAL TIME: 50 MINUTES

Any dish that combines bacon and cheese is a favorite around my house. This classic quiche is an excellent entrée for Sunday brunch that freezes well after being sliced.

Cooking spray for pie pan

1 pound thick-cut bacon, grease reserved

1 tablespoon minced garlic

¼ cup minced onion

4 eggs, beaten

1½ cups heavy (whipping) cream

1 cup shredded Swiss cheese

½ cup shredded Gruyère cheese

¾ teaspoon salt

¼ teaspoon freshly ground black pepper

PER SERVING
(⅛ OF QUICHE)
RATIO: 4:1
CALORIES: 498
TOTAL FAT: 42.7g
CARBS: 2.3g
NET CARBS: 2.3g
FIBER: 0g
PROTEIN: 22.1g

1. Preheat the oven to 350°F.

2. Lightly spray the pie pan. In a large skillet over medium-high heat, cook the bacon until crispy, 6 to 8 minutes depending on thickness. Remove the bacon from the skillet to drain on paper towels, reserving the remaining bacon grease in the skillet. Once cooled, chop the bacon into small pieces and set aside.

3. To the remaining grease in the skillet with the heat lowered to medium, add the minced garlic and onions. Cook for 3 to 4 minutes, browning slightly. Remove the skillet from the heat. Spoon the onion and garlic mixture into a small bowl. Set aside to cool.

4. In a large bowl, beat the eggs and heavy cream with a whisk for 2 minutes to combine.

5. Add the Swiss and Gruyère cheeses, reserved bacon, onions and garlic, salt, and pepper to the eggs. Whisk to combine.

6. Slowly pour the egg mixture into the prepared pie pan.

7. Carefully place the pan on the middle rack in the oven. Bake for 20 to 25 minutes, until the center has solidified.

8. Remove the pan from the oven. Cool the quiche for 5 minutes before slicing and serving.

BROCCOLI AND CHEESE QUICHE CUPS

MAKES 4 QUICHE CUPS
PREP TIME: 10 MINUTES ■ COOK TIME: 35 MINUTES ■ TOTAL TIME: 45 MINUTES

Light, fluffy eggs pair with sharp Cheddar cheese and broccoli in this simple breakfast dish. Enjoy this recipe using ramekins for individual servings. They make a great lunch accompanied by a side salad.

Cooking spray for ramekins

½ teaspoon salt, plus additional for salting the cooking water

1½ cups broccoli florets

5 eggs

¾ cup heavy (whipping) cream

¼ teaspoon freshly ground black pepper

½ teaspoon minced garlic

¾ cup shredded sharp Cheddar cheese

1. Preheat the oven to 350°F.

2. Spray four ramekins with cooking spray and place them on a baking sheet.

3. Bring a medium pot of salted water to a boil. Add the broccoli. Cook for 1 minute. Drain the broccoli from the pot. Transfer to paper towels to finish draining.

4. Chop the drained broccoli. Set aside.

5. In a large bowl, whisk together the eggs, heavy cream, salt, and pepper. Fold in the broccoli, garlic, and cheese.

6. Divide the egg mixture evenly among the prepared ramekins. Place the baking sheet with the ramekins into the preheated oven.

7. Bake until the egg and broccoli mixture has risen and is slightly browned, about 35 minutes.

COOKING TIP: Save time by buying broccoli steamer bags and popping them in the microwave. You can prep the other ingredients at the same time, and it will save on dirty dishes.

BACON & BEYOND BREAKFAST

PER SERVING
(1 QUICHE CUP)
RATIO: 3:1
CALORIES: 255
TOTAL FAT: 21.1g
CARBS: 3.8g
NET CARBS: 2.7g
FIBER: 0.9g
PROTEIN: 13.7g

CHEESY AVOCADO BAKED EGGS

SERVES 2

PREP TIME: 10 MINUTES • COOK TIME: 20 MINUTES • TOTAL TIME: 30 MINUTES

A healthy, quick, and easy way to start your day, baked eggs in avocado halves offer endless ways to experiment. Try them with a variety of cheeses, toppings, and seasonings like chopped onion and chives, or cayenne pepper and hot sauce.

1 avocado, halved lengthwise, pitted

2 eggs

4 tablespoons shredded Colby cheese, divided

⅛ teaspoon salt, divided

⅛ teaspoon freshly ground black pepper, divided

BACON & BEYOND BREAKFAST

PER SERVING (1 AVOCADO HALF WITH EGG AND CHEESE FILLING)

RATIO: 4:1

CALORIES: 324

TOTAL FAT: 28.5g

CARBS: 9.5g

NET CARBS: 2.7g

FIBER: 6.8g

PROTEIN: 10.8g

1. Preheat the oven to 475°F.

2. Scoop out enough avocado from each half so an egg fits. Place each avocado half in a ramekin, setting it into the ramekin, cut side facing up.

3. Using two small bowls, carefully crack an egg into each. Do not break the yolk.

4. Spoon one yolk into each avocado half and fill to the brim with egg white.

5. Sprinkle 2 tablespoons of Colby cheese over each avocado half. Season evenly with the salt and pepper.

6. Place the ramekins in the preheated oven carefully so the avocado halves don't tip over.

7. Bake 15 to 20 minutes, or to your desired doneness.

BACON-WRAPPED ASPARAGUS AND EGGS

SERVES 2

PREP TIME: 10 MINUTES ▪ COOK TIME: 20 MINUTES ▪ TOTAL TIME: 30 MINUTES

This sumptuous breakfast is my personal go-to for a lazy Saturday morning when I'm craving something out of the ordinary. Asparagus wrapped in bacon accompanies runny fried eggs to create a unique combination in this dish. I like to enjoy it with a dollop of sour cream or crème fraîche for additional fat.

4 bacon slices

12 asparagus spears, divided

1 teaspoon minced garlic

½ teaspoon onion powder

½ teaspoon salt, divided

¼ teaspoon freshly ground black pepper, divided

1 tablespoon butter

4 eggs

PER SERVING (2 EGGS WITH 2 BACON-WRAPPED ASPARAGUS BUNDLES)

RATIO: 3:1

CALORIES: 479

TOTAL FAT: 35.5g

CARBS: 8.3g

NET CARBS: 5.1g

FIBER: 3.2g

PROTEIN: 32.9g

1. Preheat the oven to 400°F.

2. Wrap one bacon slice around each bundle of three asparagus spears. Place each bundle on a parchment-lined baking sheet.

3. Sprinkle the garlic, onion powder, ¼ teaspoon of salt, and a pinch of pepper over the bundles.

4. Place the tray in the preheated oven. Bake for 12 minutes, or until the bacon crisps.

5. In a large skillet over medium-high heat, melt the butter. Crack the eggs in pairs into the skillet. Try to keep the yolks intact.

6. Cook the eggs to your desired doneness, about 5 minutes for a runny egg. Season with the remaining ¼ teaspoon of salt and the remaining pepper.

7. Remove the asparagus from the oven.

8. Remove the eggs from the skillet, placing two eggs atop two bundles of asparagus per serving.

SCOTCH EGGS

SERVES 2

PREP TIME: 15 MINUTES • COOK TIME: 25 MINUTES • TOTAL TIME: 45 MINUTES

Easy to make and enjoy today or save for later and reheat, scotch eggs are a versatile and compact breakfast. The type of breakfast sausage you choose will largely determine how the final meal will taste. Be aware that the thickness of the sausage patties around the eggs can alter the cooking time.

½ cup breakfast sausage

½ teaspoon garlic powder

¼ teaspoon salt

⅛ teaspoon freshly ground black pepper

2 hardboiled eggs, peeled

PER SERVING
(1 SAUSAGE-
WRAPPED EGG)

RATIO: 3:1

CALORIES: 258

TOTAL FAT: 20.5g

CARBS: 1g

NET CARBS: 1g

FIBER: 0g

PROTEIN: 16.7g

1. Preheat the oven to 400°F.

2. In a medium bowl, mix together the sausage, garlic powder, salt, and pepper. Shape the sausage into two balls.

3. On a piece of parchment paper, flatten each ball into a ¼-inch-thick patty.

4. Place one hardboiled egg in the center of each patty and gently shape the sausage around the egg.

5. Place the sausage-covered eggs on an ungreased baking sheet and into the preheated oven.

6. Bake for 25 minutes. Allow 5 minutes to cool, and then serve.

EGGS BENEDICT

SERVES 2
PREP TIME: 10 MINUTES · COOK TIME: 10 MINUTES · TOTAL TIME: 20 MINUTES

Another breakfast classic you're able to enjoy on keto is Eggs Benedict. Instead of an English muffin, substitute a layer of bacon for the necessary crunch. If your hollandaise sauce gets too thick while it rests, simply add a few drops of warm water and mix before serving.

FOR THE HOLLANDAISE SAUCE

2 eggs

1½ teaspoons freshly squeezed lemon juice

¼ cup butter, melted

¼ teaspoon salt

FOR THE EGGS

4 slices bacon

1 teaspoon vinegar

4 eggs

PER SERVING
(2 EGGS, 2 BACON
SLICES, ½ OF THE
HOLLANDAISE
SAUCE)

RATIO: 3:1

CALORIES: 624

TOTAL FAT: 53.9g

CARBS: 1.8g

NET CARBS: 1.8g

FIBER: 0g

PROTEIN: 32.6g

To make the hollandaise sauce

1. In a large heat-safe bowl, whisk two eggs and the lemon juice together vigorously until thick and almost double in volume.

2. Fill a large skillet with 1 inch of water and heat to simmering. Reduce the heat to medium.

3. Wearing a heat-resistant oven glove, hold the bowl with the eggs over the water, making sure it does not touch the water. Whisk the mixture for about 3 minutes, being careful not to scramble the eggs.

4. Slowly add the butter to the egg mixture and continue to whisk until it thickens, about 2 minutes.

5. Whisk in the salt.

6. Refrigerate the sauce until cool.

   (continued)

To make the eggs

1. Pour the water out of the skillet and place it over medium-high heat. Place the bacon in the skillet. Cook for 3 minutes per side. Transfer the bacon to paper towels to drain.

2. In a medium saucepan half full of water, add the vinegar and bring to a low boil.

3. Gently crack the eggs into the water, being careful not to break the yolks. Reduce the heat to medium-low. Cook for 3 to 4 minutes.

4. Remove the eggs. Allow them to drain and set aside.

To assemble the finished dish

1. Break each bacon slice in half. Place two halves on a plate and top with one egg. Repeat with 2 more halves and another egg.

2. Cover with hollandaise sauce.

3. Repeat with the remaining bacon and eggs for the second serving.

DENVER OMELET

SERVES 1

PREP TIME: 10 MINUTES   COOK TIME: 5 MINUTES   TOTAL TIME: 15 MINUTES

All the way from the Mile High City, this classic omelet has all of my favorite breakfast options in one place. Vegetables, cheese, and savory meat make this a perfect keto meal for my weekday mornings, especially with sautéed garlic, which adds an additional flavor punch to the overall dish.

1 tablespoon butter

¼ cup chopped onion

¼ cup chopped red bell pepper

¼ cup chopped green bell pepper

½ teaspoon minced garlic

¼ cup diced cooked ham

2 eggs, beaten

¼ teaspoon salt

⅛ teaspoon freshly ground black pepper

¼ cup shredded Cheddar cheese

1. In a medium nonstick skillet over medium-high heat, melt the butter.

2. Add the onion, red bell pepper, green bell pepper, garlic, and ham. Sauté until the ham is crisp, about 2 minutes.

3. In a small bowl, beat the eggs with the salt and pepper. Pour the eggs into the skillet with the vegetables and ham. Reduce the heat to medium.

4. Cook the eggs for 3 to 4 minutes. Flip the omelet over. After flipping, top one-half of the omelet with the Cheddar cheese.

5. After 1 to 2 minutes, fold the omelet over, covering the cheese. Cook for another 1 to 2 minutes, until the cheese melts.

6. Remove the omelet from the skillet to a plate, and serve.

**BACON & BEYOND
BREAKFAST**

PER SERVING
(1 OMELET)

RATIO: 3:1

CALORIES: 429

TOTAL FAT: 32.7g

CARBS: 9.1g

NET CARBS: 6.9g

FIBER: 2.2g

PROTEIN: 24.7g

PORTOBELLO, SAUSAGE, AND CHEESE BREAKFAST "BURGER"

SERVES 1

PREP TIME: 5 MINUTES • COOK TIME: 20 MINUTES • TOTAL TIME: 25 MINUTES

Portable and delicious, this breakfast "burger" uses sausage instead of beef for the center patty. Enjoy this recipe with or without toppings, and don't forget to experiment to find your favorite cheese combination. It is also important to make sure your Portobello mushrooms are similar in thickness so they cook for the same amount of time.

1 tablespoon olive oil

2 Portobello mushroom caps, stemmed, gills removed

¼ cup breakfast sausage

2 (2-ounce) slices American cheese

1. In a medium nonstick skillet over medium heat, heat the olive oil for 1 minute.

2. Place the mushroom caps into the hot oil, cap side up. Cook for about 5 minutes per side, or until browned.

3. Heat another medium skillet over medium-high heat.

4. Form the breakfast sausage into a ½-inch-thick patty. Place it in the center of the heated pan. Cook for 4 to 5 minutes. Flip and cook 2 to 3 minutes more.

5. When the sausage is almost done, reduce the heat to low. Top the patty with the American cheese. Cook until the cheese melts.

6. Transfer the mushroom caps from their skillet to a plate.

7. Place the cheese-topped patty on one mushroom cap. Top with the remaining mushroom cap and serve.

BISCUITS AND SAUSAGE GRAVY

SERVES 6

PREP TIME: 20 MINUTES • COOK TIME: 30 MINUTES • TOTAL TIME: 50 MINUTES

A Southern classic, biscuits and gravy get the keto treatment in this adapted recipe. With the addition of cheese and sour cream, these biscuits develop a fluffy texture that is sure to rival your grandmother's recipe. The thick, creamy sausage gravy is the perfect companion to these delectable biscuits.

FOR THE BISCUITS

½ cup coconut flour

½ cup almond flour

2 teaspoons baking powder

1 teaspoon garlic powder

½ teaspoon onion powder

½ teaspoon salt

½ cup shredded Cheddar cheese

¼ cup butter, melted

4 eggs

¾ cup sour cream

FOR THE SAUSAGE GRAVY

1 pound ground breakfast sausage

1 teaspoon minced garlic

1 tablespoon almond flour

1½ cups unsweetened almond milk

½ cup heavy (whipping) cream

1½ teaspoons freshly ground black pepper

½ teaspoon salt

PER SERVING
(1 BISCUIT, ⅓ CUP SAUSAGE GRAVY)

RATIO: 3:1

CALORIES: 559

TOTAL FAT: 48.5g

CARBS: 14.2g

NET CARBS: 8.2g

FIBER: 6g

PROTEIN: 14.6g

To make the biscuits

1. Preheat the oven to 350°F degrees.

2. Line a baking sheet with parchment paper.

3. In a large bowl, combine the coconut flour, almond flour, baking powder, garlic powder, onion powder, and salt. Slowly incorporate the Cheddar cheese.

4. In the center of the dry ingredients, create a well for adding the wet ingredients.

5. Into this well, add the melted butter, eggs, and sour cream. Fold together until a dough forms.

6. Use a spoon to drop biscuits onto the prepared baking sheet, placing them 1 inch apart.

7. Bake the biscuits for 20 minutes, or until firm and lightly browned.

(continued)

To make the sausage gravy

1. Heat a large saucepan over medium-high heat. Add the ground sausage, breaking it up with spoon and browning it on all sides.

2. Once the sausage browns, add the minced garlic. Cook for 1 minute.

3. Once the garlic is fragrant, sprinkle in the almond flour. Reduce the heat to medium-low. Allow the almond flour to incorporate with the grease to develop a light roux, stirring constantly, about 5 minutes.

4. Slowly add the almond milk to the roux, stirring constantly.

5. Add the heavy cream. Increase the temperature to medium-high, stirring and reducing the mixture for 3 minutes.

6. Reduce the heat to medium-low. Add the pepper and salt. Stir for 1 minute to incorporate.

7. Check the biscuits and remove the baking sheet from the oven when ready. Cool the biscuits for 5 minutes.

8. Reduce the heat again under the sausage gravy to low. Simmer while the biscuits cool.

9. Once the biscuits are cool, plate 1 biscuit per person and top with ⅓ cup of gravy.

ALMOND FLOUR PANCAKES

SERVES 3

PREP TIME: 10 MINUTES • COOK TIME: 15 MINUTES • TOTAL TIME: 25 MINUTES

This thicker, heartier keto version of pancakes will fill you up quickly, and they take sugar-free maple syrup very well. The baking soda and sparkling water allow the almond flour to puff up, creating a less dense and more palatable cake. Add a pat of Cinnamon Butter (page 227) or your favorite berries for a tasty, fibrous breakfast.

1 cup almond flour

1 tablespoon stevia, or other sugar substitute

¼ teaspoon salt

1 teaspoon baking powder

2 eggs

⅛ cup heavy (whipping) cream

⅛ cup sparkling water

½ teaspoon pure vanilla extract

2 tablespoons coconut oil, melted

Cooking spray for griddle

PER SERVING
(2 PANCAKES)

RATIO: 4:1

CALORIES: 383

TOTAL FAT: 34

CARBS: 7.9g

NET CARBS: 3.9g

FIBER: 4g

PROTEIN: 3.8g

1. Preheat a griddle over medium-high heat.

2. In a large bowl, mix together the almond flour, stevia, salt, and baking powder.

3. Create a small well in the center of the dry ingredients. Add the eggs, heavy cream, sparkling water, vanilla, and coconut oil. Mix together thoroughly.

4. Spray the griddle with cooking spray. Pour the batter onto the griddle in desired amounts. Cook the pancakes for 2 to 3 minutes, until you see little bubbles, then flip. Cook for an additional 1 to 2 minutes.

5. Remove the pancakes from the griddle when done. Repeat with the remaining batter.

CREAM CHEESE PANCAKES

SERVES 1

PREP TIME: 5 MINUTES — COOK TIME: 10 MINUTES — TOTAL TIME: 15 MINUTES

These crêpe-thin pancakes make a wonderful base for your favorite breakfast toppings. Sugar-free maple syrup, Cinnamon Butter (page 227), and a touch of whipped cream make these a Saturday morning go-to. If the batter is too runny, try using a cookie cutter or similar device on the griddle to keep the batter in place.

¼ cup cream cheese, at room temperature

2 eggs

½ teaspoon stevia

¼ teaspoon nutmeg

PER SERVING
(6 TO 8 PANCAKES)
RATIO: 3:1
CALORIES: 327
TOTAL FAT: 28.7g
CARBS: 2.5g
NET CARBS: 2.5g
FIBER: 0g
PROTEIN: 15.4g

1. Heat a griddle over medium-low heat.

2. Place the cream cheese in a blender. Add the eggs, stevia, and nutmeg. Pulse until the batter is smooth.

3. Slowly pour a small amount of the batter onto the griddle, about one-eighth cup per pancake. The batter will be very thin and spread easily.

4. Cook the pancake for just over 1 minute before gently flipping. Cook for another minute before removing from the pan.

5. Repeat with the remaining batter.

WAFFLES WITH WHIPPED CREAM

MAKES 4 TO 5 WAFFLES

PREP TIME: 5 MINUTES ▪ COOK TIME: 10 MINUTES ▪ TOTAL TIME: 15 MINUTES

While waffles may be hard to replicate on the keto diet in terms of crunchiness, they are easy to match when it comes to flavor. This recipe yields a light, flavorful batter that can be adapted to your needs. For a thicker batter, use fewer egg whites.

FOR THE WAFFLES

Cooking spray for waffle iron

¼ cup coconut flour

¼ cup almond flour

¼ cup flax meal

1 teaspoon baking powder

1 teaspoon stevia, or other sugar substitute

¼ teaspoon cinnamon

¾ cup egg whites (about 3 whites)

4 whole eggs

1 teaspoon pure vanilla extract

FOR THE WHIPPED CREAM

½ cup heavy (whipping) cream

1 teaspoon stevia, or other sugar substitute

PER SERVING
(2 WAFFLES, ½ OF THE WHIPPED CREAM)

RATIO: 3:1

CALORIES: 420

TOTAL FAT: 27.1g

CARBS: 15.7g

NET CARBS: 6.5g

FIBER: 9.2g

PROTEIN: 27g

To make the waffles

1. Heat the waffle iron to medium-high heat.

2. Coat with cooking spray.

3. In a large bowl, whisk together the coconut flour, almond flour, flax meal, baking powder, stevia, and cinnamon.

4. In another medium bowl, beat the egg whites until stiff peaks form.

5. Add the whole eggs and vanilla to the dry ingredients. Mix well to combine.

6. Gently fold the beaten egg whites into the dry ingredients until fully incorporated.

7. Pour the batter onto the preheated waffle iron. Cook according to waffle iron directions.

(continued)

To make the whipped cream

1. In a medium bowl, whip the heavy cream for 3 to 4 minutes, until thick.

2. Add the stevia. Continue to whisk until stiff peaks form, about 1 minute more.

3. Top the waffles with equal amounts of the whipped cream and serve.

BACON & BEYOND
BREAKFAST

CINNAMON MUFFINS WITH CREAM CHEESE FROSTING

SERVES 12

PREP TIME: 15 MINUTES • COOK TIME: 25 MINUTES • TOTAL TIME: 50 MINUTES

These fluffy cinnamon-flavored muffins paired with cream cheese frosting will satisfy even the most intense cinnamon-roll craving. The mixture of almond and coconut flours creates the perfect texture, and the addition of sparkling water helps the batter rise while baking. Store the muffins unfrosted and, when ready to eat, warm slightly before adding the cream cheese topping.

FOR THE CINNAMON MUFFINS

1 cup almond flour

½ cup coconut flour

2 teaspoons baking powder

¼ cup erythritol, or other sugar substitute, like stevia

6 eggs

½ cup butter, melted

½ cup sparkling water

1 teaspoon pure vanilla extract

1½ tablespoons cinnamon

FOR THE CREAM CHEESE FROSTING

8 ounces (1 package) cream cheese, at room temperature

1 tablespoon sour cream

½ teaspoon pure vanilla extract

BACON & BEYOND BREAKFAST

PER SERVING
(1 MUFFIN WITH CREAM CHEESE FROSTING)

RATIO: 3:1

CALORIES: 225

TOTAL FAT: 18.5g

CARBS: 6.2g

NET CARBS: 3.1g

FIBER: 3.1g

PROTEIN: 5.3g

To make the cinnamon muffins

1. Preheat the oven to 350°F.

2. In a medium bowl, whisk together the almond flour, coconut flour, baking powder, and erythritol.

3. In a large bowl, whisk the eggs. Add the melted butter, sparkling water, and vanilla. Whisk to combine.

4. Add the dry ingredients to the wet ingredients. Mix well to combine.

5. Spoon the batter evenly into a cupcake pan. Top each muffin with an equal amount of cinnamon.

(continued)

6. Using a toothpick, swirl the cinnamon into the batter.

7. Place the cupcake pan in the preheated oven. Bake for 20 to 25 minutes, or until golden brown.

8. Remove the cupcake pan from the oven and cool the muffins in the pan for 5 to 10 minutes.

To make the cream cheese frosting

In a medium bowl, blend the cream cheese, sour cream, and vanilla. Refrigerate until needed. Distribute evenly on the muffins before serving.

BACON & BEYOND BREAKFAST

RASPBERRY SCONES

SERVES 8

PREP TIME: 10 MINUTES COOK TIME: 15 MINUTES TOTAL TIME: 35 MINUTES

Delicious on their own or paired with Cinnamon Butter (page 227), these scones make for a great quick breakfast that will satisfy your morning baked-goods cravings. The addition of berries gives these scones an added nutrient boost. If raspberries are not in season, use any other berry you like.

1 cup almond flour

2 eggs, beaten

⅓ cup Splenda, stevia, or other sugar substitute

1½ teaspoons pure vanilla extract

1½ teaspoons baking powder

½ cup raspberries

1. Preheat the oven to 375°F.

2. Line a baking sheet with parchment paper.

3. In a large bowl, combine the almond flour, eggs, Splenda, vanilla, and baking powder. Mix well.

4. Add the raspberries to the bowl and gently fold in.

5. After the raspberries are incorporated, spoon 2 to 3 tablespoons of the batter, per scone, onto the parchment-lined baking sheet.

6. Place the baking sheet into the preheated oven. Bake for 15 minutes, or until lightly browned.

7. Remove the baking sheet from the oven. Place the scones on a rack to cool for 10 minutes.

INGREDIENT TIP: Depending on the size of the raspberries, you may want to cut your berries in halves or quarters before adding to the batter. Doing this spreads the raspberry flavor throughout the scone.

BACON & BEYOND BREAKFAST

PER SERVING (1 SCONE)

RATIO: 3:1

CALORIES: 133

TOTAL FAT: 8.6g

CARBS: 4g

NET CARBS: 2g

FIBER: 2g

PROTEIN: 1.5 g

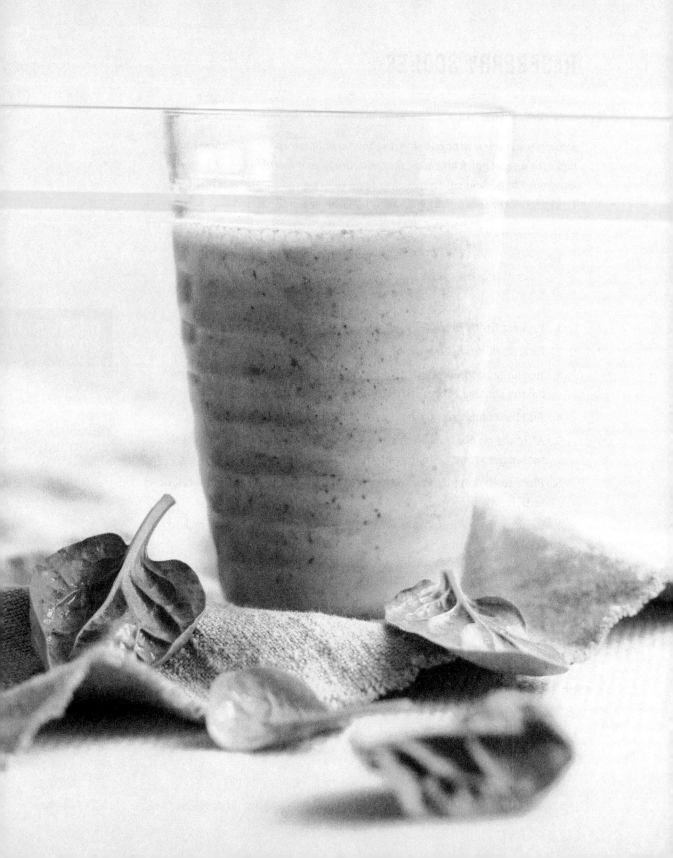

CHAPTER

3

SUPER RICH SMOOTHIES & SHAKES

TRIPLE BERRY SMOOTHIE

SERVES 2

TOTAL TIME: 10 MINUTES

All of my favorite berries come together in this super fruity and fibrous smoothie. This tall glass of refreshment was a staple meal for me during busy workdays, often replacing lunch. Since berries tend to be high in fiber they are lower on the glycemic index scale, making them a great superfood for anyone on the keto diet. Enjoy this smoothie with fresh or frozen berries, depending on the time of year.

1 cup crushed ice, divided

½ cup unsweetened almond milk

1 tablespoon coconut oil

½ cup blueberries

½ cup raspberries

½ cup blackberries

½ teaspoon pure vanilla extract

PER SERVING
(½ OF FINISHED
SMOOTHIE RECIPE)

RATIO: 3:1

CALORIES: 252

TOTAL FAT: 21.6g

CARBS: 15.8g

NET CARBS: 9.7g

FIBER: 6.1g

PROTEIN: 2.5g

1. In a blender, place ½ cup of ice. Add the almond milk and coconut oil. Blend to combine.

2. Add the blueberries, raspberries, blackberries, vanilla, and remaining ½ cup of ice.

3. Blend for 1 minute, or until smooth, and serve.

MEAN GREEN SMOOTHIE

SERVES 2
TOTAL TIME: 10 MINUTES

Boasting three types of leafy greens, this epic smoothie is perfect for an early morning boost or midday snack. Filled with kale, spinach, and Swiss chard, it provides nutrients like iron, magnesium, calcium, and vitamin C—all of which are necessary for a healthy mind and body. Add herbs like parsley or cilantro for an extra flavor bite.

1½ cups crushed ice, divided

1 cup kale, tightly packed, cleaned, stalks removed

½ cup spinach, cleaned, stalks removed

½ cup Swiss chard, cleaned, stalks removed

2 tablespoons coconut oil

2 tablespoons chia seeds

½ cup water

1. In a blender, place ¾ cup of ice. Add the kale, spinach, and Swiss chard. Blend to combine.

2. Add the coconut oil, chia seeds, remaining ¾ cup of ice, and water.

3. Blend for 1 minute, or until smooth, and serve.

COOKING TIP: Save time on this recipe by using prewashed frozen spinach, kale, and—if available—Swiss chard. If using frozen vegetables, reduce the ice in this recipe by ¼ cup.

PER SERVING
(½ OF FINISHED
SMOOTHIE RECIPE)
RATIO: 3:1
CALORIES: 293
TOTAL FAT: 23.3g
CARBS: 14.6g
NET CARBS: 3.4g
FIBER: 11.2g
PROTEIN: 7.7g

STRAWBERRY SPINACH SMOOTHIE

SERVES 2

TOTAL TIME: 10 MINUTES

Strawberry and spinach may sound like an odd combination but they come together in an amazing way in this unique recipe. (Have you ever enjoyed strawberries in your spinach salad?) If strawberries are not in season, don't hesitate to use frozen strawberries. They're usually picked and frozen fresh at the peak of the season. Frozen spinach is also an option, though fresh is preferred for its bright flavor.

1 cup crushed ice, divided

½ cup unsweetened almond milk

2 cups fresh spinach

½ cup strawberries

1 tablespoon coconut oil

1. In a blender, place ½ cup of ice. Add the almond milk, spinach, strawberries, and coconut oil. Blend to combine.

2. Add the remaining ½ cup of ice.

3. Blend for 1 minute, or until smooth, and serve.

GREEN TEA SMOOTHIE

SERVES 2
TOTAL TIME: 10 MINUTES

Packed with an energizing kick, this green tea smoothie will wake you up on even the foggiest of days. Green tea powder isn't just an energizer; it's also full of fiber and nutrients like vitamin C, selenium, zinc, and magnesium. Experiment with the amount of green tea powder, as you desire.

1 cup crushed ice, divided

1 cup unsweetened almond milk

¼ cup heavy (whipping) cream

1 tablespoon coconut oil

3 tablespoons unsweetened vanilla protein powder

1½ teaspoons green tea powder

1. In a blender, place ½ cup of ice. Add the almond milk, heavy cream, and coconut oil. Blend to combine.
2. Add the vanilla protein powder, green tea powder, and remaining ½ cup of ice.
3. Blend for 1 minute, or until smooth, and serve.

SUPER RICH SMOOTHIES & SHAKES

PER SERVING
(½ OF FINISHED SMOOTHIE RECIPE)
RATIO: 4:1
CALORIES: 442
TOTAL FAT: 41g
CARBS: 7.3g
NET CARBS: 4.2g
FIBER: 2.9g
PROTEIN: 16.6g

COCONUT BERRY SMOOTHIE

SERVES 2

TOTAL TIME: 10 MINUTES

Like a blast of the tropics, this coconut berry smoothie is rich with bursts of flavor from blackberries and raspberries while still smooth and creamy from the coconut milk. Raspberries and blackberries are an excellent source of vitamin C and are high in fiber, which makes this a heart-healthy recipe, too. Since coconut milk comes in a variety of options, always look for full-fat coconut milk and stock up when you can.

1 cup crushed ice, divided

1 cup unsweetened, full-fat coconut milk

1 tablespoon coconut oil

½ cup raspberries

½ cup blackberries

2 tablespoons unsweetened coconut flakes

PER SERVING
(½ OF FINISHED
SMOOTHIE RECIPE)

RATIO: 4:1

CALORIES: 384

TOTAL FAT: 37.5g

CARBS: 14.5g

NET CARBS: 7.5g

FIBER: 7g

PROTEIN: 3.8g

1. In a blender, place ½ cup of ice. Add the coconut milk and coconut oil. Blend to combine.

2. Add the raspberries, blackberries, coconut flakes, and remaining ½ cup of ice.

3. Blend for 1 minute, or until smooth, and serve.

FRUGAL FRIENDLY TIP: Save money on pricey unsweetened coconut flakes by buying in bulk and freezing batches ready for use. Coconut keeps very well in the freezer, but do not freeze it in its original packaging, which may not be appropriate for freezer storage. Instead, transfer to a zip-top freezer bag.

AVOCADO COCONUT SMOOTHIE

SERVES 2
TOTAL TIME: 10 MINUTES

Creamy avocado blends with thick coconut milk in this unique but extremely filling smoothie. Similar in texture, avocado and coconut go very well together. Their flavors meld and are accented by the coconut flakes in this recipe for an extra coco-nutty kick.

1 cup crushed ice, divided

1 avocado, peeled and pitted

1 cup unsweetened, full-fat coconut milk

1 tablespoon coconut oil

1 tablespoon unsweetened coconut flakes

1. In a blender, place ½ cup of ice. Add the avocado, coconut milk, and coconut oil. Blend to combine.
2. Add the remaining ½ cup of ice and coconut flakes.
3. Blend for 1 minute, or until smooth, and serve.

SUPER RICH SMOOTHIES & SHAKES

PER SERVING
(½ OF FINISHED
SMOOTHIE RECIPE)
RATIO: 4:1
CALORIES: 512
TOTAL FAT: 51.2g
CARBS: 13g
NET CARBS: 6g
FIBER: 7g
PROTEIN: 4g

AVOCADO BLUEBERRY SMOOTHIE

SERVES 2

TOTAL TIME: 10 MINUTES

Creamy avocado blends with bursts of blueberry in this delicious smoothie that's perfect as a meal replacement on the go. The bright flavor of the blueberry complements the silky texture of the avocado for a truly unique treat. Use frozen blueberries unless they are in peak season to ensure the freshest fruit quality.

1 cup crushed ice, divided

½ cup blueberries

¾ cup unsweetened almond milk

2 tablespoons heavy (whipping) cream

1 tablespoon coconut oil

1 avocado, peeled and pitted

1. In a blender, place ½ cup of ice. Add the blueberries, almond milk, heavy cream, and coconut oil. Blend to combine.

2. Add the avocado and remaining ½ cup of ice.

3. Blend for 1 minute, or until smooth, and serve.

INGREDIENT VARIATION: Try this smoothie with blackberries instead of blueberries for a different twist on the berry and avocado pairing. Blackberries have a distinct flavor, and a smoother, more velvety texture than blueberries.

PER SERVING
(½ OF FINISHED
SMOOTHIE RECIPE)

RATIO: 4:1

CALORIES: 543

TOTAL FAT: 53.5g

CARBS: 0.9g

NET CARBS: 0.9g

FIBER: 0g

PROTEIN: 1.3g

ALMOND KALE SMOOTHIE

SERVES 2
TOTAL TIME: 10 MINUTES

The rich, savory flavor of kale pairs with the light sweetness of almonds in this recipe. Kale is a supercharged vegetable, full of vitamin C and vitamin A, both of which are important for general health. Almonds are a keto-favorite food due to their high-fat but low-protein content.

1 cup crushed ice, divided

1 cup unsweetened almond milk

1 cup kale

1 tablespoon coconut oil

2 tablespoons almond flour

½ teaspoon almond extract

1. In a blender, place ½ cup of ice. Add the almond milk, kale, and coconut oil. Blend to combine.
2. Add the almond flour, almond extract, and remaining ½ cup of ice.
3. Blend for 1 minute, or until smooth, and serve.

SUPER RICH SMOOTHIES & SHAKES

PER SERVING
(½ OF FINISHED SMOOTHIE RECIPE)
RATIO: 4:1
CALORIES: 396
TOTAL FAT: 39.2g
CARBS: 11.4g
NET CARBS: 7.5g
FIBER: 3.9g
PROTEIN: 3.8g

PEANUT BUTTER SHAKE

SERVES 2
TOTAL TIME: 10 MINUTES

Thick, creamy, and peanut buttery, this shake will keep you full for hours. The powdered peanut butter lets you control the carbohydrates in this recipe, as most jarred peanut butters are sugar-sweetened. If you have unsweetened peanut butter, feel free to substitute that for the powdered peanut butter and coconut oil.

1 cup crushed ice, divided

¼ cup powdered peanut butter (such as PB2)

¼ cup heavy (whipping) cream

2 tablespoons coconut oil

1 cup unsweetened almond milk

1. In a blender, place ½ cup of ice. Add the powdered peanut butter and heavy cream. Blend to combine.
2. Add the coconut oil, almond milk, and remaining ½ cup of ice.
3. Blend for 1 minute, or until smooth, and serve.

PER SERVING
(½ OF FINISHED
SMOOTHIE RECIPE)
RATIO: 4:1
CALORIES: 535
TOTAL FAT: 50.8g
CARBS: 17.1g
NET CARBS: 10.5g
FIBER: 6.6g
PROTEIN: 13.1g

DOUBLE CHOCOLATE SHAKE

SERVES 2
TOTAL TIME: 10 MINUTES

Almond milk mixes with cocoa powder and dark-chocolate chunks to create a double-chocolate treat in this luscious shake. Crumbly chocolate chunks are definitely a treat, and should be high quality (90 to 100 percent cacao). If you're looking for a pick-me-up after a long day, this is it.

1 cup crushed ice, divided

¾ cup unsweetened almond milk

¼ cup heavy (whipping) cream

1 tablespoon coconut oil

3 tablespoons unsweetened chocolate protein powder

1 tablespoon unsweetened cocoa powder

1 tablespoon chopped 90 percent dark chocolate

1 tablespoon sugar-free chocolate syrup

1. In a blender, place ½ cup of ice. Add the almond milk, heavy cream, and coconut oil. Blend to combine.

2. Add the protein powder, cocoa powder, dark chocolate, chocolate syrup, and remaining ½ cup of ice.

3. Blend for 1 minute, or until smooth, and serve.

SUPER RICH SMOOTHIES & SHAKES

PER SERVING
(½ OF FINISHED SMOOTHIE RECIPE)
RATIO: 4:1
CALORIES: 451
TOTAL FAT: 41g
CARBS: 19g
NET CARBS: 13.3g
FIBER: 5.7g
PROTEIN: 9.8g

STRAWBERRIES AND CREAM SHAKE

SERVES 2
TOTAL TIME: 10 MINUTES

Strawberries and cream on a diet may seem like a stretch, but not on keto. Mixed with lots of dairy fats, this recipe relies on the simplicity of its ingredients to let the flavor of the strawberries shine through. For more of a strawberry flavor, look for a sugar-free strawberry syrup to add to the mix.

1 cup crushed ice, divided

¼ cup unsweetened almond milk

½ cup heavy (whipping) cream

1 tablespoon coconut oil

½ cup strawberries

1 teaspoon pure vanilla extract

1. In a blender, place ½ cup of ice. Add the almond milk, heavy cream, and coconut oil. Blend to combine.
2. Add the strawberries, vanilla, and remaining ½ cup of ice.
3. Blend for 1 minute, or until smooth, and serve.

PER SERVING
(½ OF FINISHED
SMOOTHIE RECIPE)
RATIO: 4:1
CALORIES: 249
TOTAL FAT: 25.2g
CARBS: 5.5g
NET CARBS: 4.1g
FIBER: 1.4g
PROTEIN: 1.6g

CHOCOLATE, PEANUT BUTTER, AND BANANA SHAKE

SERVES 2
TOTAL TIME: 10 MINUTES

I like to call this one the "Elvis." This is my favorite shake to make when I'm craving sweets, or on a special morning when I feel like treating myself. Since bananas are not allowed on keto, this recipe uses banana extract. Add more for heightened banana flavor, as desired.

1 cup crushed ice, divided

3 tablespoons unsweetened chocolate protein powder

1 tablespoon unsweetened peanut butter

1 tablespoon coconut oil

1½ teaspoons cocoa powder

1 cup unsweetened almond milk

¼ cup heavy (whipping) cream

1 teaspoon banana extract

½ teaspoon pure vanilla extract

1. In a blender, place ½ cup of ice. Add the protein powder, peanut butter, and coconut oil. Blend to combine.

2. Add the cocoa powder, almond milk, heavy cream, banana extract, vanilla, and remaining ½ cup of ice.

3. Blend for 1 minute, or until smooth, and serve.

SUPER RICH SMOOTHIES & SHAKES

PER SERVING
(½ OF FINISHED SMOOTHIE RECIPE)

RATIO: 4:1

CALORIES: 473

TOTAL FAT: 45.5g

CARBS: 10.8g

NET CARBS: 7.1g

FIBER: 3.7g

PROTEIN: 10.3g

BUTTERED COFFEE SHAKE

SERVES 1

TOTAL TIME: 10 MINUTES

This colder, frostier version of Buttered Coffee (page 32) is just as good as its hot, early morning cousin. Make sure to use high-quality oil and butter to get the most benefit possible from these unique fats. Enjoy this smoothie whenever you need a boost or require mental focus.

1 cup crushed ice, divided

2 tablespoons unsalted, grass-fed butter

1½ tablespoons MCT oil, or coconut oil

1½ cups iced coffee

¼ cup heavy (whipping) cream

1. In a blender, place ½ cup of ice. Add the butter, MCT oil, and coffee. Blend to combine.

2. Add the heavy cream and remaining ½ cup of ice.

3. Blend for 1 minute, or until smooth, and serve.

SUPER RICH SMOOTHIES & SHAKES

PER SERVING
(1 RECIPE)

RATIO: 4:1

CALORIES: 486

TOTAL FAT: 54.6g

CARBS: 0.9g

NET CARBS: 0.9g

FIBER: 0g

PROTEIN: 1.3g

VANILLA SHAKE

SERVES 2
TOTAL TIME: 10 MINUTES

A true classic, this vanilla shake is made with protein powder and vanilla extract for a rich, deep flavor. Whip this shake up and add personal favorites like chopped almonds, blueberries, or cinnamon. Add extra vanilla to suit your taste.

1 cup crushed ice, divided

1 cup unsweetened almond milk

¼ cup heavy (whipping) cream

1 tablespoon coconut oil

3 tablespoons unsweetened vanilla whey protein powder

1 teaspoon pure vanilla extract

1. In a blender, place ½ cup of ice. Add the almond milk, heavy cream, and coconut oil. Blend to combine.
2. Add the protein powder, vanilla, and remaining ½ cup of ice.
3. Blend for 1 minute, or until smooth, and serve.

SUPER RICH SMOOTHIES & SHAKES

PER SERVING
(½ OF FINISHED
SMOOTHIE RECIPE)

RATIO: 4:1

CALORIES: 448

TOTAL FAT: 41g

CARBS: 7.6g

NET CARBS: 4.7g

FIBER: 2g

PROTEIN: 16.6g

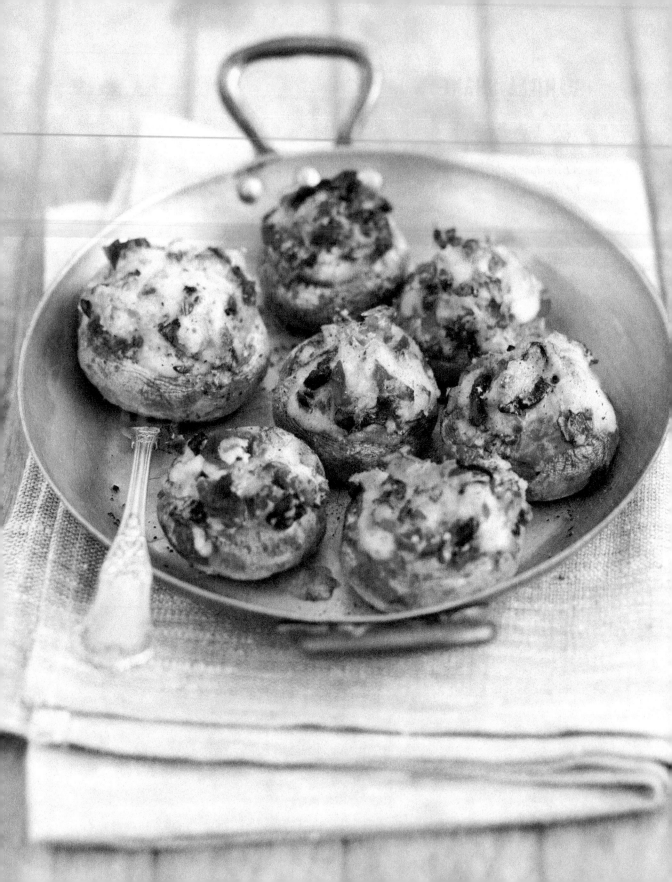

CHAPTER
4

SUMPTUOUS SNACKS

JALAPEÑO POPPERS

SERVES 1

PREP TIME: 10 MINUTES · COOK TIME: 15 MINUTES · TOTAL TIME: 25 MINUTES

When you crave something spicy, these stuffed jalapeño poppers are a great go-to snack. Depending on the time of year, jalapeños can carry a mild or medium level of heat. Paired with cream cheese, the heat is tempered but still comes through in a pleasant, tasty way.

6 jalapeño peppers

½ teaspoon minced garlic

2 tablespoons cream cheese, at room temperature

¼ teaspoon salt

⅛ teaspoon freshly ground black pepper

4 ounces Monterey Jack cheese, cubed

1 teaspoon olive oil

PER SERVING
(6 CHEESE-STUFFED
JALAPEÑOS)
RATIO: 3:1
CALORIES: 254
TOTAL FAT: 21.5g
CARBS: 7.8g
NET CARBS: 4.2g
FIBER: 3.6g
PROTEIN: 9.8g

1. Preheat the oven to 450°F.

2. Wash the jalapeños and cut off the tops. Using a small knife, cut the jalapeños top to bottom without cutting through to the other side. Gently open the peppers and remove the seeds and veins. Set the peppers aside.

3. To a small bowl, add the minced garlic, cream cheese, salt, and pepper. Mix well to combine.

4. Stuff the jalapeños with the Monterey Jack cheese so they are full but will still close.

5. With a small spoon or knife, spread an equal amount of cream cheese inside each jalapeño, over the Monterey Jack, to help bind the pepper together. Close the peppers and place them on a baking sheet.

6. Drizzle the jalapeños with olive oil and place the baking sheet in the preheated oven.

7. Bake for 15 minutes, or until browned.

INGREDIENT TIP: The oils in jalapeños can be burning and irritating. Wear protective gloves when handling them and be careful not to touch your face or other areas with sensitive skin.

BACON DEVILED EGGS

SERVES 4

PREP TIME: 5 MINUTES ▪ COOK TIME: 15 MINUTES ▪ TOTAL TIME: 20 MINUTES

A meaty twist on a classic party dish, these deviled eggs topped with bacon are an easy snack to whip up on a weekend. Prepared for you or for visiting friends, this recipe works for keto and non-keto dieters alike. Add a dash of cayenne for a spicy kick.

6 eggs

3 to 4 bacon slices (½ cup when chopped, depending on thickness)

1½ tablespoons mayonnaise

1 tablespoon mustard

½ teaspoon paprika, divided

⅛ teaspoon salt

⅛ teaspoon freshly ground black pepper

PER SERVING (3 STUFFED EGG HALVES)

RATIO: 3:1

CALORIES: 283

TOTAL FAT: 21.1g

CARBS: 3.4g

NET CARBS: 2.9g

FIBER: 0.5g

PROTEIN: 19.6g

1. Bring a large pot half filled with water to a boil. Gently place the eggs in the water, being careful not to crack the shells. Cook for 10 minutes. Remove the pot from the water. Set aside to cool.

2. While the eggs cook, heat a large skillet over medium-high heat. Add the bacon to the skillet. Cook for 3 minutes. Flip and cook for 2 to 3 minutes more, or until crisp. Transfer the bacon to paper towels to drain.

3. Once the eggs cool, gently crack the shells and peel them. Cut the peeled eggs in half lengthwise.

4. Scoop the yolks into a medium bowl. Add the mayonnaise, mustard, ¼ teaspoon paprika, salt, and pepper. Stir to combine.

5. Chop the bacon into small pieces. Divide into two equal amounts (about ¼ cup each). Add ¼ cup of bacon to the yolks. Mix well to combine.

6. Place the egg whites cut-side up on a plate. Spoon an equal amount of the yolk mixture into each.

7. Use the remaining ¼ cup of bacon and ¼ teaspoon of paprika to garnish the eggs, and serve.

COOKING TIP: Save time on this recipe by purchasing precooked bacon. While freshly cooked bacon is always preferred, buying precooked makes this recipe much quicker on those early weekday mornings.

BLACK FOREST HAM, CHEESE, AND CHIVE ROLL-UPS

SERVES 2

TOTAL TIME: 10 MINUTES

For a quick weekday snack, look no further than these Black Forest ham and cheese roll-ups. Whether you like to eat them whole or cut them into slices for a bite-size treat, they are a simple keto staple that you can vary to your liking. Try combinations like turkey and Cheddar, or roast beef and Havarti.

6 slices Black Forest ham (about 5 ounces total)

3 ounces cream cheese, at room temperature

1 tablespoon chopped fresh chives

¼ cup shredded Monterey Jack cheese

½ teaspoon garlic powder

½ teaspoon onion powder

⅛ teaspoon salt

⅛ teaspoon freshly ground black pepper

SUMPTUOUS SNACKS

PER SERVING
(3 ROLL-UPS)

RATIO: 3:1

CALORIES: 345

TOTAL FAT: 26.5g

CARBS: 5.7

NET CARBS: 4.4g

FIBER: 1.3g

PROTEIN: 21.1g

1. On a cutting board, lay out the six ham slices. Spread ½ ounce of cream cheese on each ham slice, covering evenly.

2. Distribute the chives evenly over each piece of ham.

3. Top evenly with the Monterey Jack cheese. Sprinkle each piece with the garlic powder, onion powder, salt, and pepper.

4. Roll up each slice and enjoy. If desired, slice each roll crosswise into 1-inch pieces, and serve.

BACON GUACAMOLE

SERVES 4

PREP TIME: 5 MINUTES ▪ COOK TIME: 10 MINUTES ▪ TOTAL TIME: 15 MINUTES

Watch out: This guacamole packs a punch, and not just because of the bacon. The subtle but spicy flavor from the serrano peppers is sure to tickle taste buds and delight spice lovers. If you don't want a spicy guacamole, simply omit the serrano and enjoy it without.

4 bacon slices

2 avocados, peeled, pitted, and diced

½ cup chopped yellow onion

⅓ cup chopped tomato

2 teaspoons minced garlic

1 jalapeño pepper, minced

1 serrano pepper, minced

1 tablespoon chopped fresh cilantro

1 teaspoon freshly squeezed lime juice

¼ teaspoon salt

⅛ teaspoon freshly ground black pepper

¼ teaspoon cayenne pepper

PER SERVING

RATIO: 4:1

CALORIES: 259

TOTAL FAT: 22.8g

CARBS: 11.6g

NET CARBS: 4.1

FIBER: 7.5g

PROTEIN: 5.1g

1. Heat a large skillet over medium-high heat. Add the bacon. Cook for 3 minutes. Flip and cook for another 2 to 3 minutes. Transfer the cooked bacon to paper towels to cool. Once cooled, chop the bacon and set aside.

2. In a large bowl, combine the avocados, onion, and tomato.

3. Add the garlic, jalapeño pepper, and serrano pepper. Gently fold the ingredients together.

4. Before the ingredients are fully incorporated, add the cilantro, chopped bacon, lime juice, salt, black pepper, and cayenne pepper to the bowl. Mix all ingredients together. Do not overmix.

5. Serve immediately.

BUFFALO CHICKEN DIP

SERVES 8

PREP TIME: 10 MINUTES COOK TIME: 40 MINUTES TOTAL TIME: 55 MINUTES

If Sundays at your house are reserved for football like they are at mine, this dip is sure to be a touchdown hit for the whole crowd. Packed with cheesy goodness and spicy chicken, this recipe will have you scraping the edges to get every last bite. I like to tone the heat up with some heavy-handed shakes of hot sauce—my favorite is Tabasco Chipotle Pepper Sauce for a light smoky flavor.

½ cup butter

1 teaspoon minced garlic

4 boneless chicken thighs

¼ cup sour cream

¼ teaspoon salt

¼ teaspoon freshly ground black pepper

¼ teaspoon cayenne pepper

¼ teaspoon paprika

8 ounces (1 package) cream cheese, at room temperature

½ cup hot sauce, additional as needed

½ cup Ranch Dressing (page 218), or purchased bottled dressing

1 cup shredded mozzarella cheese

½ cup shredded Cheddar cheese

1. Preheat the oven to 450°F.

2. Heat a large skillet with a cover over medium-high heat. Add the butter and melt.

3. Add the garlic and chicken to the skillet. Cook for 3 minutes. Reduce the heat to medium. Turn the chicken so it cooks on all sides, cooking for 12 to 15 minutes total.

4. With a meat thermometer, check the chicken for doneness. It should reach 165°F. When cooked, remove the chicken to a large bowl. Set aside to cool.

5. Shred the cooled chicken into bite-size pieces.

6. Add the sour cream, salt, black pepper, cayenne pepper, and paprika to the shredded chicken. Mix well.

7. In a 9-inch-square pan, spread the cream cheese over the bottom and up the sides, coating evenly. Pour the chicken mixture over the cream cheese layer.

8. Drizzle the hot sauce and Ranch Dressing over the chicken mixture, distributing evenly.

9. Top with the mozzarella and Cheddar cheeses.

10. Using a butter knife, swirl the ingredients together in the pan.

11. Place the pan in the preheated oven. Bake for 15 minutes, or until the top layer is browned and bubbling.

12. Remove the pan from the oven. Cool the dip for 5 minutes before serving.

INGREDIENT TIP: Add crumbled bacon or bleu cheese to take this dip to the next level. This recipe can also be made with chicken breasts if you do not have chicken thighs (though the dark meat of the thighs does lend additional flavor to the overall dish).

FRIED AVOCADO

SERVES 3

PREP TIME: 5 MINUTES   COOK TIME: 10 MINUTES   TOTAL TIME: 17 MINUTES

These fried avocado wedges are an absolute delight. Crispy and crunchy on the outside, and soft and creamy on the inside, they're always a hit and can be seasoned in a variety of ways. Dip them in Ranch Dressing (page 218) for some added flavor.

Oil for frying

1 egg

1 tablespoon heavy (whipping) cream

1 avocado, peeled and pitted

¼ teaspoon salt

¼ teaspoon freshly ground black pepper

¼ cup shredded Parmesan cheese

¼ cup pork rinds, ground

¼ teaspoon onion powder

¼ teaspoon garlic powder

1. Fill a large, deep skillet with about 1½ inches of oil. Preheat the oil to 375°F.

2. In a small bowl, create an egg wash by whisking together the egg and heavy cream.

3. Cut the avocado into ½-inch-thick slices. Season with the salt and pepper.

4. On a medium plate, mix together the Parmesan cheese, pork rinds, onion powder, and garlic powder.

5. Dip each avocado slice in the egg wash, drain off the excess, and then dip into the pork rind coating, covering completely.

6. Once the oil is hot, slowly drop in the avocado slices a few at a time. Fry for 1 to 2 minutes, or until golden brown. Remove the slices and set aside on paper towels to drain. Repeat with the remaining slices.

7. Cool for 1 to 2 minutes before serving.

CRISPY KALE CHIPS

SERVES 2

PREP TIME: 5 MINUTES ▪ COOK TIME: 25 MINUTES ▪ TOTAL TIME: 33 MINUTES

This recipe is delicious as well as nutritious. Enjoy these chips with a quick dip in some Ranch Dressing (page 218) or on their own as a filling snack. Keep an eye on these while they're baking—they can burn very quickly.

2 cups kale, cleaned, leaves trimmed from stalk

1 tablespoon olive oil

½ teaspoon salt

½ teaspoon freshly ground black pepper

½ teaspoon onion powder

½ teaspoon garlic powder

1. Preheat the oven to 300°F.
2. In a large bowl, add kale leaves and the olive oil. Toss to coat the leaves evenly with the oil.
3. Add the salt, pepper, onion powder, and garlic powder to the bowl. Toss again to coat the leaves evenly.
4. On a parchment-lined baking sheet, spread the kale into an even layer. Place the sheet in the preheated oven.
5. Bake for 10 minutes, rotate the baking sheet, then bake for an additional 15 minutes.
6. Remove the baking sheet from the oven. Cool the kale on the tray for 3 minutes before serving.

COOKING TIP: If you have an oil-dispensing spray can, use it on these kale chips. Too much oil will weigh them down, causing them to burn instead of crisp, and too little oil will leave them wilted. The ability to coat each leaf evenly makes a big difference.

PER SERVING

RATIO: 3:1

CALORIES: 99

TOTAL FAT: 7g

CARBS: 8.3g

NET CARBS: 7.2g

FIBER: 1.2g

PROTEIN: 2.2g

BUFFALO ROASTED CAULIFLOWER WITH BLEU CHEESE SAUCE

SERVES 3

PREP TIME: 5 MINUTES • COOK TIME: 20 MINUTES • TOTAL TIME: 27 MINUTES

This is the perfect snack when you are craving the flavor of buffalo wings but don't want to deal with the hassle of making them. Cauliflower is an amazing, incredibly versatile vegetable that is able to take on many flavors. Try this recipe with other marinades and sauces, like fajita mix and sour cream.

FOR THE ROASTED CAULIFLOWER

2 cups cauliflower florets

1 tablespoon olive oil

1 teaspoon garlic powder

1 teaspoon onion powder

¼ teaspoon salt

⅛ teaspoon freshly ground black pepper

FOR THE BUFFALO SAUCE

¼ cup butter

⅓ cup hot sauce

1 tablespoon white vinegar

¼ teaspoon Worcestershire sauce

FOR THE BLEU CHEESE SAUCE

2 tablespoons bleu cheese dressing

2 tablespoons sour cream

⅛ cup crumbled bleu cheese

PER SERVING

RATIO: 4:1

CALORIES: 340

TOTAL FAT: 33.1g

CARBS: 6.4g

NET CARBS: 4.3g

FIBER: 1.9 g

PROTEIN: 6.5g

To make the roasted cauliflower

1. Preheat the oven to 425°F.

2. In a large bowl, combine the cauliflower florets, olive oil, garlic powder, onion powder, salt, and pepper. Mix well to season evenly.

3. On a parchment-lined baking sheet, spread the cauliflower into an even layer. Bake for 20 minutes, or until the edges of the cauliflower pieces begin to brown.

To make the buffalo sauce

1. In a large skillet over medium-high heat, add the butter and melt.

2. Add the hot sauce, vinegar, and Worcestershire sauce. Whisk over medium-high heat until the mixture is bubbling. Remove the skillet from the heat.

To make the bleu cheese sauce

In a small bowl, whisk together the bleu cheese dressing and sour cream. Fold in the crumbled bleu cheese. Cover and refrigerate until ready to serve.

To make the finished dish

In a large bowl, toss the cooked cauliflower with the buffalo sauce to coat. Allow the cauliflower to cool for 1 to 2 minutes before serving with the bleu cheese sauce.

INGREDIENT TIP: Add cayenne pepper for an extra kick, or pick an extra-spicy hot sauce to create your buffalo sauce. Be careful if you start cutting up peppers. The capsaicin, which gives the peppers their heat, will stay on your fingers and can burn. Always wear gloves when chopping hot peppers and remember to wash your hands thoroughly immediately after handling the peppers. Also, be careful not to touch your hands to your face or any other area with sensitive skin.

ROSEMARY ROASTED ALMONDS

SERVES 4

PREP TIME: 5 MINUTES   COOK TIME: 15 MINUTES   TOTAL TIME: 20 MINUTES

Full of fresh rosemary flavor, this simple snack is a personal and party favorite at my home. Fresh rosemary is key here, so save this recipe for another time if you only have dried rosemary on hand. I fell so in love with the flavor of these that I now keep a small rosemary bush on the back porch. Enjoy these nuts with a cup of tea or alongside cured meats and cheeses.

1½ cups almonds

1 tablespoon olive oil

1 tablespoon chopped fresh rosemary

½ teaspoon salt

½ teaspoon freshly ground black pepper

¼ teaspoon ground ginger

PER SERVING
(½ CUP)
RATIO: 4:1
CALORIES: 240
TOTAL FAT: 21.5g
CARBS: 8.4g
NET CARBS: 3.5g
FIBER: 4.9g
PROTEIN: 7.6g

1. Preheat the oven to 325°F.

2. In a medium bowl, combine the almonds and olive oil. Mix until the almonds are evenly coated.

3. Add the rosemary, salt, pepper, and ginger to the almonds. Stir to combine.

4. On a baking sheet covered with aluminum foil, spread the almonds into an even layer. Place the sheet in the preheated oven.

5. Bake for 15 minutes, or until toasted.

FRUGAL FRIENDLY TIP: Almonds are often less expensive per pound when purchased in bulk. Look for bulk dry goods sections at your grocery store or visit a store like Costco for the best deals.

PROSCIUTTO AND CREAM CHEESE STUFFED MUSHROOMS

SERVES 4

PREP TIME: 5 MINUTES ▪ COOK TIME: 20 MINUTES ▪ TOTAL TIME: 27 MINUTES

Perfect for a party appetizer or an afternoon snack, these stuffed mushrooms roasted with cream cheese and prosciutto are a lovely treat. Prosciutto comes in a variety of thicknesses; for this recipe, the thinner the better. When prosciutto is cooked it can become tough if it's too thick, so ask your butcher for the thinnest cut available.

¾ cup cream cheese, at room temperature

¼ cup sour cream

4 slices prosciutto, chopped

1 teaspoon chopped fresh parsley

¼ teaspoon salt

⅛ teaspoon freshly ground black pepper

16 small button mushrooms, stemmed, gills removed

1 tablespoon olive oil

PER SERVING (4 STUFFED MUSHROOMS)

RATIO: 4:1

CALORIES: 279

TOTAL FAT: 25g

CARBS: 3.1g

NET CARBS: 2.6g

FIBER: 0.5g

PROTEIN: 12g

1. Preheat the oven to 400°F.

2. In a large bowl, mix together the cream cheese and sour cream. Add the prosciutto, parsley, salt, and pepper. Stir to combine.

3. Spoon equal amounts of the cream cheese and prosciutto mixture into the mushrooms.

4. On a parchment-lined baking sheet, arrange the mushrooms, cream-cheese-side up. Drizzle with the olive oil. Bake for 20 minutes, or until slightly browned.

5. Remove the baking sheet from the oven. Cool for 1 to 2 minutes before serving.

ZUCCHINI MINI PIZZAS

SERVES 2

PREP TIME: 10 MINUTES ■ COOK TIME: 5 MINUTES ■ TOTAL TIME: 15 MINUTES

Sometimes you just want pizza. For a quick snack, nothing could be easier than these Zucchini Mini Pizzas. Sprinkled with mozzarella cheese and topped with pepperoni, these tasty treats will have you thinking about making another batch before you're even done with the first.

1 medium zucchini, sliced diagonally (about 8 slices)

1 teaspoon olive oil

2 tablespoons sugar-free pizza sauce

¼ cup shredded mozzarella cheese

¼ cup goat cheese, crumbled

16 pepperoni slices (optional)

⅛ teaspoon salt

⅛ teaspoon freshly ground black pepper

1 teaspoon Italian seasoning

PER SERVING
(4 MINI PIZZAS)
RATIO: 3:1
CALORIES: 220
TOTAL FAT: 15.9g
CARBS: 6.6g
NET CARBS: 4.2g
FIBER: 1.4g
PROTEIN: 14.1g

1. Preheat the oven to broil.

2. Place the zucchini slices on a baking sheet and drizzle with the olive oil.

3. Broil the zucchini for 2 minutes per side. Remove the baking sheet from the oven.

4. Top each slice with equal amounts of the pizza sauce, mozzarella cheese, and goat cheese.

5. Top each with two slice of pepperoni (if using).

6. Season each slice evenly with the salt, pepper, and Italian seasoning.

7. Place the baking sheet back in the oven. Broil for 2 minutes, or until the cheese browns.

SPINACH AND ARTICHOKE DIP

SERVES 8

PREP TIME: 5 MINUTES ▪ COOK TIME: 25 MINUTES ▪ TOTAL TIME: 35 MINUTES

A favorite of many, spinach and artichoke dip is the perfect thing to scoop up with some pork rinds for a tasty snack. Although this dip is traditionally made with mozzarella and Parmesan, this recipe includes the rich, nutty flavor of Gruyère for added cheesiness.

2 tablespoons butter

2 tablespoons minced garlic

1¼ cups spinach, chopped

1¾ cups artichoke hearts, chopped

8 ounces (1 package) cream cheese

1 cup Parmesan cheese, divided

½ cup shredded mozzarella cheese

½ cup shredded Gruyère cheese

3 tablespoons sour cream

1 tablespoon mayonnaise

½ teaspoon salt

½ teaspoon freshly ground black pepper

½ teaspoon paprika

PER SERVING
RATIO: 3:1
CALORIES: 259
TOTAL FAT: 20.3g
CARBS: 9.4g
NET CARBS: 5.8g
FIBER: 3.6g
PROTEIN: 12.5g

1. Preheat the oven to 375°F.

2. In a large skillet over medium-high heat, melt the butter. Add the garlic. Cook for 1 minute. Add the chopped spinach and cook for 1 to 2 minutes more. Add the artichokes and cook for an additional minute. Transfer the spinach and artichoke mixture to a large bowl.

3. Reduce the heat under the skillet to medium-low. Add the cream cheese to the pan. Melt until creamy.

4. Add ½ cup of Parmesan cheese, the mozzarella cheese, and the Gruyère cheese. Stir until the cheeses melt, about 2 minutes.

5. Pour the melted cheeses over the spinach and artichoke mixture. Stir to combine.

6. Add the sour cream, mayonnaise, salt, pepper, and paprika. Stir to incorporate.

7. Transfer the spinach and artichoke mixture to a 9-inch-square pan. Sprinkle with the remaining ½ cup of Parmesan cheese.

8. Bake for 20 to 25 minutes, or until the top is browned and bubbling.

9. Cool the dip for 5 minutes before serving.

CHEESE CRACKERS

SERVES 2

PREP TIME: 5 MINUTES   COOK TIME: 15 MINUTES   TOTAL TIME: 35 MINUTES

When you're craving a crunchy snack, these cheese crackers will surprise you with their crisp texture and rich flavor. While Cheddar is used in this recipe, other semi-hard cheeses, like Parmesan, work equally well. Enjoy these with a light dip or your favorite toppings.

8 tablespoons shredded Cheddar cheese

1. Preheat the oven to 375°F.
2. On a parchment-lined baking sheet, spoon the cheese by tablespoons into eight piles, spaced at least 1½ inches apart.
3. Place the sheet in the preheated oven. Bake for 10 to 15 minutes, until golden brown.
4. Remove the sheet from the oven. Cool the crackers on the sheet for 10 to 15 minutes.
5. Gently remove each cracker from the parchment and enjoy.

PERFECT PAIRING: Try these with French Onion Dip (page 88) for a burst of oniony flavor alongside the crispness of the cheese. They are also great with a scoop of Buffalo Chicken Dip (page 76) on top.

SUMPTUOUS SNACKS

PER SERVING
(4 CRACKERS)
RATIO: 3:1
CALORIES: 114
TOTAL FAT: 9.4g
CARBS: 0.4g
NET CARBS: 0.4g
FIBER: 0g
PROTEIN: 7g

GOAT CHEESE STUFFED ROASTED PEPPERS

SERVES 4

PREP TIME: 10 MINUTES ▪ COOK TIME: 15 MINUTES ▪ TOTAL TIME: 25 MINUTES

Treat yourself to a tapas classic with these goat cheese stuffed peppers, roasted to perfection. The rich, creamy flavor of the goat cheese cuts through the light spice of the pepper and is complemented by the fresh basil. If you are unable to find fresh basil, make this recipe when you have it, as dried basil does not produce the same flavors when used as a substitute.

¾ cup goat cheese, at room temperature

1 teaspoon minced garlic

2 teaspoons chopped fresh basil

¼ teaspoon salt

⅛ teaspoon freshly ground black pepper

12 sweet cherry peppers, stemmed and seeded

1 tablespoon olive oil

1. Preheat the oven to 425°F.

2. In a small bowl, mix together the goat cheese, garlic, basil, salt, and pepper.

3. With a spoon, fill the peppers with the goat cheese mixture.

4. Place the peppers on a parchment-lined baking sheet. Drizzle the peppers with the olive oil. Put the baking sheet in the oven.

5. Bake for 15 minutes, or until the peppers are browned and the cheese is bubbling.

SUMPTUOUS SNACKS

PER SERVING
(3 STUFFED PEPPERS)
RATIO: 3:1
CALORIES: 253
TOTAL FAT: 18.6g
CARBS: 5.1g
NET CARBS: 3.1g
FIBER: 2g
PROTEIN: 13g

FRENCH ONION DIP

SERVES 4

PREP TIME: 5 MINUTES   COOK TIME: 45 MINUTES   TOTAL TIME: 2 HOURS

While you may buy French onion dip at the store, this recipe will make you quickly reconsider that decision. Caramelizing onions does bring out the sugars more but this dip can be enjoyed in moderation on the keto diet. Paired with pork rinds or raw vegetables, this dip can be enjoyed right after you make it or after resting in the refrigerator overnight for enhanced flavor.

2 tablespoons butter

1½ cups chopped yellow onion

¾ teaspoon salt, divided

1 cup sour cream

½ cup mayonnaise

1 teaspoon minced garlic

1 teaspoon Worcestershire sauce

½ teaspoon freshly ground black pepper

SUMPTUOUS
SNACKS

PER SERVING

RATIO: 3:1

CALORIES: 207

TOTAL FAT: 18.4g

CARBS: 9.4g

NET CARBS: 8.4g

FIBER: 1g

PROTEIN: 1.7g

1. In a large skillet over medium-high heat, melt the butter. Add the onions and ¼ teaspoon of salt. Cook for 1 to 2 minutes. Reduce the heat to medium-low. Allow the onions to caramelize for 35 to 40 minutes, stirring occasionally.

2. Remove the onions from the heat. Allow them to cool while preparing the remaining ingredients.

3. In a medium bowl, mix together the sour cream, mayonnaise, garlic, Worcestershire sauce, pepper, and remaining ½ teaspoon of salt.

4. Add the cooled onions to the mixture. Stir to combine.

5. Before serving, cover and refrigerate the dip for 1 hour to allow the flavors to meld, or overnight for the best-tasting results.

CHEESY PORK RIND NACHOS

SERVES 1

PREP TIME: 10 MINUTES ■ COOK TIME: 5 MINUTES ■ TOTAL TIME: 15 MINUTES

Though tortilla chips are nowhere to be found on the keto diet, you can still enjoy nachos with the crunchy, salty flavor of pork rinds. Serving as the base for just about any type of nacho you can think of, this basic cheese recipe can be built on with your keto favorites. For a spicy kick, try pickled jalapeños.

1½ ounces pork rinds

⅓ cup shredded Mexican cheese blend

⅛ cup diced tomato

1 garlic clove, minced

¼ teaspoon cumin

⅛ cup sour cream

Fresh cilantro for garnish

1. Arrange the pork rinds on a large microwaveable plate, being careful not to overlap them.

2. Sprinkle the cheese evenly over all the pork rinds, covering each one to the edges.

3. Top with the tomatoes and garlic. Season with the cumin.

4. Place the plate in a microwave. Cook on high for 1 minute, 15 seconds. Check to see if the cheese has melted. If needed, cook for another 15 to 30 seconds, checking frequently. Make sure not to overcook, or the pork rinds will become soggy.

5. Remove the plate from the microwave. Garnish the nachos with sour cream and cilantro. Serve.

SUMPTUOUS SNACKS

PER SERVING

RATIO: 3:1

CALORIES: 461

TOTAL FAT: 33.4g

CARBS: 4.5g

NET CARBS: 4.5g

FIBER: 0g

PROTEIN: 36.7g

BACON-WRAPPED MOZZARELLA STICKS

SERVES 2

PREP TIME: 10 MINUTES · COOK TIME: 5 MINUTES · TOTAL TIME: 15 MINUTES

Gooey mozzarella cheese is encased in bacon, a keto staple, in this favorite snack recipe. In Sneaky Keto Classics (chapter 5), you'll find a recipe for a more traditional style of mozzarella sticks, but since everything is better with bacon, why not give these a try? Crunchy on the outside but melty on the inside, these are a crowd pleaser as well as an indulgent late-night snack.

Oil for frying

2 mozzarella string cheese pieces

4 bacon slices

PER SERVING
(2 BACON-WRAPPED
CHEESE STICKS)
RATIO: 3:1
CALORIES: 381
TOTAL FAT: 29.3g
CARBS: 1.7g
NET CARBS: 1.7g
FIBER: 0g
PROTEIN: 27.5g

1. In a large saucepan, heat 2 inches of oil to 350°F.

2. Cut each string cheese stick in half widthwise.

3. Wrap each half of string cheese in one slice of bacon. Secure with a toothpick. Keep the ends of the cheese stick exposed for better cooking.

4. Once the oil is hot, drop the bacon-wrapped cheese pieces into the oil. Cook for 2 to 3 minutes, or until the bacon is thoroughly browned. Transfer to paper towels to drain.

5. Serve alone or with sugar-free marinara sauce.

CAPRESE SALAD BITES

SERVES 6
TOTAL TIME: 15 MINUTES

Perfect for a party or a quick midday snack, these Caprese Salad Bites are full of flavor and simple to make. The bright burst of flavor from the tomato pairs perfectly with the creamy mozzarella and fresh basil. Drizzled with olive oil, these little skewers get a zing from balsamic vinegar and a simple seasoning of salt and pepper for a well-rounded bite.

12 cherry tomatoes, halved

12 bocconcini (small mozzarella balls), or 12 (1-ounce) mozzarella cubes

12 fresh basil leaves

2 tablespoons olive oil

1 tablespoon balsamic vinegar

¼ teaspoon salt

⅛ teaspoon freshly ground black pepper

1. Using a toothpick, spear one tomato half, then add one bocconcini.

2. Top the cheese with one basil leaf then the second tomato half. Set aside.

3. Repeat the process with the remaining ingredients.

4. Arrange the skewered bites on a tray. Drizzle with the olive oil and balsamic vinegar. Season with the salt and pepper.

5. Serve immediately, or chill for up to 24 hours.

PER SERVING
(2 SALAD BITES)
RATIO: 3:1
CALORIES: 287
TOTAL FAT: 19.4g
CARBS: 8.3g
NET CARBS: 5.3g
FIBER: 3g
PROTEIN: 16.4g

GARLIC PEPPERONI CHIPS

SERVES 4

PREP TIME: 5 MINUTES ・ COOK TIME: 10 MINUTES ・ TOTAL TIME: 15 MINUTES

Whenever a potato chip craving hits, I reach for this meaty and delicious recipe to satisfy it. Pepperoni is high in fat content, which allows it to crisp up in the oven. Be careful, though; one minute too long and these chips will go from perfection to a burned mess very quickly. I've had plenty of smoke alarm run-ins trying to perfect these crunchy delights.

6 ounces pepperoni slices

½ teaspoon garlic powder

SUMPTUOUS SNACKS

PER SERVING
(1½ OUNCES
PEPPERONI)

RATIO: 4:1

CALORIES: 200

TOTAL FAT: 17g

CARBS: 0.2g

NET CARBS: 0.2g

FIBER: 0g

PROTEIN: 8.6g

1. Preheat the oven to 425°F.

2. On a parchment-lined baking sheet, lay out the pepperoni slices about ½ inch apart.

3. Sprinkle the slices with the garlic powder.

4. Place the sheet in the preheated oven. Bake for 7 to 8 minutes. Remove the tray and flip each slice.

5. Return the tray to the oven. Bake for another 2 to 3 minutes, or until the pepperoni slices are golden brown and crispy. Remove the sheet from the oven and transfer the slices to a plate lined with paper towels to dry.

6. Store in an airtight container for up to 2 days.

HOT DOG ROLLS

SERVES 4

PREP TIME: 10 MINUTES ▪ COOK TIME: 15 MINUTES ▪ TOTAL TIME: 30 MINUTES

Hot dogs without the bun are always great for a quick keto meal, but these fast and easy Hot Dog Rolls are also perfect for on-the-go eating. Made with a cheesy, almond-flour crust, they puff up a lot while baking but their texture is perfectly bready when done. Dip these in sugar-free marinara, or omit the Italian seasoning and pair with Sugar-Free Ketchup (page 216) and mustard for a ballpark feel.

1½ cups shredded mozzarella cheese

2 tablespoons cream cheese, at room temperature

¾ cup almond flour

1 egg

1 teaspoon minced garlic

1 teaspoon Italian seasoning

4 hot dogs

1. Preheat the oven to 425°F.

2. In a large microwaveable bowl, combine the mozzarella cheese and cream cheese. Microwave on high for 1 minute. Remove, stir, and microwave again for 30 seconds more. The mixture will be very hot.

3. Add the almond flour, egg, garlic, and Italian seasoning to the cheese mixture. Stir to incorporate fully.

4. With wet hands, divide the dough into four equal pieces. Shape one piece of dough around each hot dog, encasing the hot dog completely.

5. Place the dough-wrapped hot dogs onto a parchment-lined baking sheet. Use a fork to poke holes into each piece of dough so it doesn't bubble up during cooking.

6. Put the baking sheet into the preheated oven. Bake for 7 to 8 minutes.

7. Remove the tray from the oven. Check for bubbles (prick with a fork, if formed). Turn the dogs over. Return to the oven for another 6 to 7 minutes.

8. Remove the sheet from the oven. Cool the hot dog rolls for 3 to 5 minutes before serving.

SUMPTUOUS SNACKS

PER SERVING
(1 HOT DOG ROLL)

RATIO: 4:1

CALORIES: 435

TOTAL FAT: 34.7g

CARBS: 7.6g

NET CARBS: 5.3g

FIBER: 2.3g

PROTEIN: 18.6g

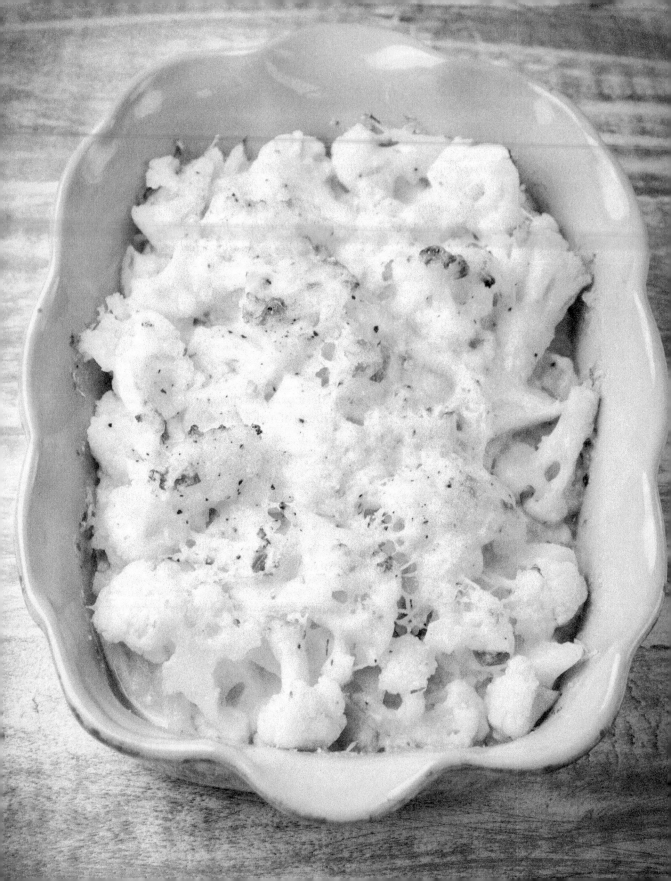

CHAPTER
5

SNEAKY KETO
CLASSICS

CAULIFLOWER MAC AND CHEESE

SERVES 8

PREP TIME: 10 MINUTES — COOK TIME: 30 MINUTES — TOTAL TIME: 45 MINUTES

Cauliflower is an extremely versatile vegetable, especially on the keto diet. It can take on many forms and flavors, which makes it the perfect carbohydrate substitute. In this recipe, cauliflower pairs with a rich, creamy cheese sauce that will curb any pasta craving. This recipe was one of the first that I tested when starting keto, and it is an incredibly easy way to develop a love for the lifestyle. My friends beg for this dish when they come over for dinner—it's that good!

1 teaspoon salt, divided

1 head fresh cauliflower, chopped into small florets

1 cup heavy (whipping) cream

⅓ cup cream cheese, cubed

1 cup shredded Cheddar cheese

½ cup shredded mozzarella cheese

½ teaspoon minced garlic

¼ teaspoon freshly ground black pepper

Cooking spray for baking pan

½ cup shredded Parmesan cheese

PER SERVING

RATIO: 3:1

CALORIES: 198

TOTAL FAT: 16.8g

CARBS: 3.3g

NET CARBS: 2.4g

FIBER: 0.9g

PROTEIN: 9.6g

1. Preheat the oven to 400°F.

2. Bring a large pot of water to a boil. Season with ½ teaspoon of salt. Carefully drop the cauliflower into the boiling water and cook for 5 minutes. Drain thoroughly, and place the florets on paper towels to soak up any remaining moisture. Put the cauliflower in a large bowl and set aside.

3. To a large skillet over medium heat, add the heavy cream and bring to a simmer. Whisk in the cream cheese until smooth. Add the Cheddar cheese, mozzarella cheese, and garlic. Whisk until the cheeses melt, about 2 minutes.

4. Remove the cheese sauce from heat and pour over the cauliflower. Stir to coat the florets evenly. Sprinkle with the remaining ½ teaspoon of salt and the pepper.

5. Spray an 8-inch-square baking pan with cooking spray. Transfer the cauliflower mixture to the pan. Top with the Parmesan cheese.

6. Place the pan in the preheated oven. Bake for 20 minutes, or until the top is browned.

7. Cool for 5 minutes before serving.

COOKING TIP: Save time by microwaving a bag of packaged cauliflower florets (fresh or frozen). If you are substituting bagged cauliflower, use 2½ to 3 cups of florets in this recipe.

CAULIFLOWER "RICE"

SERVES 6

PREP TIME: 5 MINUTES ▪ COOK TIME: 15 MINUTES ▪ TOTAL TIME: 20 MINUTES

In addition to being a great pasta substitute, cauliflower is excellent as "rice," as well. You may not even be able to tell the difference in a stir-fry or when it is served with a flaky piece of fish. Fresh cauliflower is key for this recipe, so save the bagged cauliflower for other recipes.

1 head fresh cauliflower, florets removed
and stalk discarded

1. Preheat the oven to 425°F.

2. In the bowl of a food processor, place the cauliflower and pulse for about 1 minute, or until the cauliflower is in very small pieces.

3. Set aside any cauliflower "rice" you do not plan to use immediately. It freezes well in resealable bags.

4. Spread the remaining cauliflower evenly on a baking sheet. Place the sheet in the preheated oven. Bake for 7 minutes. Remove the sheet from the oven, stir, and flip the cauliflower. Return the sheet to the oven for another 7 to 8 minutes.

5. When finished, use in a stir-fry or serve as a dish on its own.

SNEAKY KETO
CLASSICS

PER SERVING
RATIO: 3:1
CALORIES: 11
TOTAL FAT: 0g
CARBS: 2.3g
NET CARBS: 1.2g
FIBER: 1.1g
PROTEIN: 0.9g

PERFECT PAIR TIP: Try this Cauliflower "Rice" with the Shrimp, Bamboo Shoot, and Broccoli Stir-Fry (page 124) or the Roasted Cod with Garlic Butter and Bok Choy (page 135). Both recipes will be complemented by the "rice," which can be dressed up to suit the main dish's needs.

CAULIFLOWER MASH

SERVES 6

PREP TIME: 5 MINUTES ■ COOK TIME: 10 MINUTES ■ TOTAL TIME: 15 MINUTES

Mashed potatoes are a staple food missed frequently by many on the keto diet. Fear not, for the magic of cauliflower strikes again in this delicious Cauliflower Mash recipe, which provides a perfect way to sneak vegetables into your diet while enjoying something that feels indulgent. Add bacon bits, chives, and Cheddar cheese on top to recreate a loaded baked potato.

3 cups cauliflower florets

6 tablespoons butter

4 tablespoons grated Parmesan cheese

2 tablespoons sour cream

2 tablespoons cream cheese

2 tablespoons heavy (whipping) cream

1 teaspoon minced garlic

1 teaspoon salt

½ teaspoon freshly ground black pepper

PER SERVING

RATIO: 4:1

CALORIES: 214

TOTAL FAT: 19.5g

CARBS: 4g

NET CARBS: 2.7g

FIBER: 1.3g

PROTEIN: 7.7g

1. Bring a large pot of water to a rolling boil. Add the cauliflower florets. Cook for 4 to 5 minutes. Drain the cooked cauliflower, pressing out any excess moisture.

2. In the bowl of a food processor, combine the cauliflower florets, butter, Parmesan cheese, sour cream, cream cheese, heavy cream, garlic, salt, and pepper.

3. Pulse to combine and mix until smooth.

CAULIFLOWER TORTILLAS

SERVES 6

PREP TIME: 10 MINUTES ▪ COOK TIME: 20 MINUTES ▪ TOTAL TIME: 30 MINUTES

Is there anything that cauliflower can't replicate? It would seem not, based on the versatility of this incredible vegetable. Enjoy these cauliflower tortillas with your favorite fajita meat or pulled pork. They also serve as a great wrap for breakfast scrambles to eat on the go.

¾ head fresh cauliflower

2 eggs

½ teaspoon salt

¼ teaspoon freshly ground black pepper

PER SERVING
(1 TORTILLA)
RATIO: 3:1
CALORIES: 38
TOTAL FAT: 1.5g
CARBS: 3.7g
NET CARBS: 2g
FIBER: 1.7g
PROTEIN: 3.2g

1. Preheat the oven to 375°F.

2. To the bowl of a food processor, add the cauliflower and pulse into very fine pieces.

3. In a large microwaveable bowl, microwave the prepared cauliflower on high, about 5 minutes. Stir the cauliflower and microwave for 2 minutes more. Stir it again.

4. Using a dish towel or cheesecloth, drain all the excess water from the cauliflower.

5. Return the cauliflower to the bowl. Add the eggs, salt, and pepper. Mix well to combine.

6. On a parchment-lined baking sheet, use your hands to spread the mixture into 6 or 7 small circles, flattening them gently.

7. Place the sheet into the preheated oven. Bake for 10 minutes.

8. Remove the sheet from the oven. Carefully remove the cauliflower tortillas from the parchment and flip them. Return the tortillas to the oven and bake for 6 to 7 minutes more.

9. Crisp, as needed, in a lightly oiled skillet before serving.

INGREDIENT TIP: If you have premade Cauliflower "Rice" (page 98), use this instead and pulse a little longer to get the finer consistency. This should yield about 2 cups of riced cauliflower.

CAULIFLOWER PIZZA

SERVES 2

PREP TIME: 10 MINUTES ⬝ COOK TIME: 30 MINUTES ⬝ TOTAL TIME: 40 MINUTES

You can do almost anything with cauliflower on the keto diet. It's capable of substituting for pasta, rice, and pizza crust. In this recipe, cauliflower is paired with cheese as a binder to create a well-textured crust for a basic pizza.

FOR THE CRUST

¾ teaspoon salt, divided

2 cups cauliflower florets

1 egg

2½ cups shredded mozzarella cheese, divided

½ teaspoon garlic powder

⅛ teaspoon freshly ground black pepper

FOR THE PIZZA

¼ cup sugar-free pizza sauce, divided

10 pepperoni slices, divided

PER SERVING
(18-INCH PIZZA)

RATIO: 3:1

CALORIES: 457

TOTAL FAT: 30.7g

CARBS: 10.9g

NET CARBS: 8.6g

FIBER: 2.3g

PROTEIN: 35.5g

To make the crust

1. Preheat the oven to 450°F.

2. Bring a large pot of water to a boil. Season with ½ teaspoon of salt. Carefully drop the cauliflower into the boiling water. Cook for 8 minutes. Drain thoroughly, using paper towels to soak up any excess moisture.

3. Place the drained cauliflower into a food processor. Pulse for 1 minute until the cauliflower is "riced."

4. Transfer the cauliflower to a large bowl. Add the egg, 1 cup of mozzarella cheese, the garlic powder, the remaining ¼ teaspoon of salt, and pepper. Stir until the cheese fully melts.

5. Separate the cauliflower dough into two equal balls.

6. On a parchment-lined baking sheet, spread each ball into an 8-inch crust. The crust should be very thin.

7. Place the crusts in the preheated oven. Bake for 15 to 20 minutes, or until browned. The edges of the crust should almost be burned.

8. Remove the crusts from the oven. Turn the oven to broil.

   (continued)

To make the pizza

1. Spread ⅛ cup of pizza sauce over each crust.

2. Top each crust with ¾ cup of mozzarella cheese and half the pepperoni.

3. Return the sheet to the oven. Bake the pizzas for 2 to 3 minutes, or until the cheese is melted and bubbling.

4. Remove the sheet from the oven and allow the pizzas to cool for 3 to 5 minutes before slicing and serving.

SNEAKY KETO
CLASSICS

CHEESY-CRUST PIZZA

SERVES 4

PREP TIME: 10 MINUTES   COOK TIME: 20 TO 25 MINUTES   TOTAL TIME: 40 MINUTES

If you need a pizza crust that will make everyone in the family happy, try this crispy Cheesy-Crust Pizza made with cheese only. Bound together with an egg, the cheese crisps thoroughly before any toppings are added. If you like a lot of toppings on your pizza, try the Cauliflower Pizza recipe (page 101).

1½ cups shredded mozzarella cheese, divided

½ cup Cheddar cheese

1 egg

½ teaspoon garlic powder

¼ teaspoon salt

⅛ teaspoon freshly ground black pepper

¼ cup sugar-free pizza sauce

20 pepperoni slices

1. Preheat the oven to 450°F.

2. In a large bowl, mix 1 cup of mozzarella cheese, the Cheddar cheese, egg, garlic powder, salt, and pepper.

3. On a parchment-lined 16-inch pizza pan, spread the cheese dough evenly around the pan. The crust should be thin, but without any holes.

4. Place the pan in the oven. Bake the crust for 15 to 20 minutes, or until browned. Check the oven after 10 minutes to make sure it's not burning.

5. Remove the crust from the oven. Turn the oven to broil.

6. With paper towels, blot any excess grease from the crust.

7. Spread the sauce over the crust. Top with the remaining ½ cup of mozzarella cheese and the pepperoni.

8. Return the pan to the oven. Bake for 3 to 4 minutes, or until the cheese is melted and bubbling.

9. Remove the pan from the oven. Cool the pizza for 3 to 5 minutes before slicing and serving.

SNEAKY KETO CLASSICS

PER SERVING
(¼ OF 16-INCH PIZZA)

RATIO: 3:1

CALORIES: 351

TOTAL FAT: 26.6g

CARBS: 3.8g

NET CARBS: 3.8g

FIBER: 0g

PROTEIN: 24g

ALMOND BUTTER BREAD

SERVES 12

PREP TIME: 15 MINUTES • COOK TIME: 30 TO 40 MINUTES • TOTAL TIME: 1 HOUR

For a quick, less-complicated bread recipe, try this almond butter–based one. With only five ingredients, it's very simple to whip up in a pinch. This recipe can be finicky, so if it needs more than the recommended time in the oven to set, don't panic. At such a low oven temperature it's possible to have fluctuations in cooking time.

½ cup unflavored, unsweetened whey protein powder

⅛ teaspoon salt

2 teaspoons baking powder

½ cup unsweetened almond butter

4 eggs

1 tablespoon butter for loaf pan

PER SERVING
(1 SLICE)
RATIO: 3:1
CALORIES: 102
TOTAL FAT: 7.6g
CARBS: 2.8g
NET CARBS: 2.4g
FIBER: 0.4g
PROTEIN: 6.5g

1. Heat the oven to 300°F.

2. In a small bowl, whisk together the whey, salt, and baking powder.

3. In a large bowl, use an electric mixer to whip the almond butter until creamy. Add one egg at a time, beating well after each addition. Beat the batter until fluffy.

4. Fold the whey mixture into the almond batter. Mix gently until smooth.

5. Grease the inside of a loaf pan with the tablespoon of butter by rubbing it along the walls and into each corner.

6. Transfer the mixture to the loaf pan. Place it in the preheated oven. Bake for 30 to 40 minutes, or until the center is set.

7. Remove from the oven. Cool the loaf for 5 to 10 minutes. Run a knife along the inside edges of the pan to loosen the loaf, and tip the pan upside down to remove it. Place the loaf on a cooling rack to cool completely, about 5 minutes more.

8. Slice the bread, as needed, and refrigerate covered in plastic wrap.

COCONUT ALMOND FLOUR BREAD

SERVES 12

PREP TIME: 15 MINUTES ▪ COOK TIME: 1 HOUR ▪ TOTAL TIME: 1½ HOURS

Bread is pretty hard to come by on the keto diet, but not when you get a little creative. This nut-based bread recipe yields a fluffy, thick loaf that's perfect for sandwiches or enjoyed with a thick pat of butter. Don't omit the cooling time or the loaf will fall.

10 tablespoons butter, melted, plus 1 tablespoon for the loaf pan

1 tablespoon honey

1½ tablespoons apple cider vinegar

8 eggs

¾ cup almond flour

¾ teaspoon baking soda

¾ teaspoon salt

⅔ cup coconut flour

PER SERVING (1 SLICE)

RATIO: 3:1

CALORIES: 213

TOTAL FAT: 17.2g

CARBS: 6.5g

NET CARBS: 3.5g

FIBER: 3g

PROTEIN: 5.1g

1. Preheat the oven to 300°F.

2. In a small bowl, mix together the butter, honey, and cider vinegar. Allow the mixture to cool.

3. In a medium bowl, whisk the eggs.

4. To the eggs, add the almond flour, butter mixture, baking soda, and salt. Mix thoroughly with a hand mixer.

5. Slowly sift the coconut flour into the bowl. Mix well to combine.

6. Grease the inside of a loaf pan with 1 tablespoon of butter by rubbing it along the walls and into each corner.

7. Transfer the mixture to the loaf pan. Place it in the preheated oven. Bake for 50 to 60 minutes, until the center is set.

8. Remove the pan from the oven. Allow it to cool for at least 15 minutes. Run a knife along the inside edges of the pan to loosen the loaf, and tip the pan upside down to remove it. Place the bread on a cooling rack to cool completely, about 5 minutes more.

9. Slice the bread into 12 slices, and refrigerate covered in plastic wrap.

CHEESY TACO SHELLS

SERVES 1

PREP TIME: 5 MINUTES ▪ COOK TIME: 5 MINUTES ▪ TOTAL TIME: 10 TO 15 MINUTES

Sometimes a keto soft taco made with a lettuce shell just won't cut it when you're looking for that outer layer of crunch. When those moments tempt you, reach for this cheesy taco shell recipe and fill it with ground beef, fajita chicken, or eggs at breakfast time. Note that different cheeses require different cooking times, so stick to the type suggested below or be prepared to increase the cook time.

½ cup shredded Mexican cheese blend, divided

¼ teaspoon garlic salt

PER SERVING
(2 SHELLS)
RATIO: 3:1
CALORIES: 246
TOTAL FAT: 19.8g
CARBS: 3.1g
NET CARBS: 3.1g
FIBER: 0g
PROTEIN: 14.2g

1. On a waxed paper plate, arrange ¼ cup of cheese so it covers the entire plate to the edges. Add the garlic salt on top.

2. Place the plate in the microwave. Heat on high for 1½ minutes, or until the cheese has melted and is brown around the edges and golden in the middle.

3. Remove the plate from the microwave. With a knife, gently remove the melted cheese disk from the plate. Drape it over the edge of a cutting board placed on its side. The cheese should be draped evenly. Allow it to set for 3 to 5 minutes before moving. Repeat with the remaining ¼ cup of cheese.

4. Fill the taco shells with any desired ingredients and enjoy.

WARNING: Be patient with these cheesy taco shells. While they may seem like they won't pull apart right out of the microwave after being browned, it is still a bubbly hot plate of cheese. Be careful before attempting to remove them from the plate, and watch your fingers as your place the cheese over its drying surface.

ZUCCHINI LASAGNA

SERVES 8

PREP TIME: 20 MINUTES • COOK TIME: 50 TO 60 MINUTES • TOTAL TIME: 1½ HOURS

In certain pasta dishes, cauliflower (amazing though it is) just isn't an option. Enter zucchini—the wonder vegetable that can be sliced and spiraled into a variety of pasta shapes to replicate your favorite meals. This lasagna recipe is extra cheesy and should cool and set longer than regular lasagna so it achieves the same texture.

2 tablespoons olive oil

1 cup chopped onion

1 teaspoon minced garlic

1 pound 75-percent lean ground beef

2 cups unsweetened pasta sauce

2 tablespoons chopped fresh oregano

¼ teaspoon salt

1 tablespoon chopped fresh basil

2 medium zucchinis, sliced lengthwise into ⅛-inch-thick slices (about 24 slices)

1 cup ricotta cheese, divided

8 tablespoons shredded mozzarella cheese, divided

½ cup shredded Parmesan cheese

¼ teaspoon freshly ground black pepper

PER SERVING (⅛ OF LASAGNA)

RATIO: 3:1

CALORIES: 345

TOTAL FAT: 20.9g

CARBS: 9.6g

NET CARBS: 6.6g

FIBER: 3g

PROTEIN: 24.7g

1. Preheat the oven to 375°F.

2. In a large saucepan over medium-high heat, heat the olive oil for about 1 minute. Add the onion and garlic. Sauté until tender, about 6 minutes.

3. Add the ground beef. Cook, breaking apart with a spoon, until browned, about 5 minutes.

4. Add the pasta sauce. Bring the mixture to a simmer. Reduce the heat to low. Add the oregano, salt, and basil. Stir to combine.

5. In an 8-inch-square baking dish, arrange 6 zucchini slices on the bottom. Pour one-quarter of the meat sauce over the zucchini. Dot with ¼ cup of ricotta cheese and 2 tablespoons of mozzarella.

6. Repeat the layering process three more times with the remaining zucchini, sauce, and cheeses, alternating the direction of the zucchini slices each time.

7. Top with the Parmesan cheese and pepper.

8. Place the dish in the preheated oven. Bake for 50 to 60 minutes, or until the top is browned and bubbling.

9. Remove from the oven. Cool for 15 minutes before slicing and serving.

SPAGHETTI SQUASH WITH MEATBALLS

SERVES 4

PREP TIME: 20 MINUTES • COOK TIME: 30 MINUTES • TOTAL TIME: 50 MINUTES

Why miss spaghetti on a low-carb diet when it still exists inside a delicious and nutritious vegetable? This recipe is full of Italian flavor from the fresh parsley, basil, and oregano. Sure to please the whole family with its hearty flavor, this meal will turn into a staple recipe in no time.

FOR THE SPAGHETTI SQUASH

1 large spaghetti squash

3 tablespoons water

2 tablespoons olive oil, divided

½ cup chopped fresh parsley, divided

FOR THE MEATBALLS

½ pound 80-percent lean ground beef

½ pound ground pork

½ cup shredded Parmesan cheese, divided

2 tablespoons chopped fresh basil

2 tablespoons chopped fresh oregano

½ teaspoon onion powder

½ teaspoon minced garlic

¼ teaspoon salt

¼ teaspoon freshly ground black pepper

1 cup sugar-free pasta sauce

SNEAKY KETO
CLASSICS

PER SERVING
(3 MEATBALLS,
¼ CUP SAUCE,
¼ OF SQUASH)

RATIO: 3:1

CALORIES: 460

TOTAL FAT: 28g

CARBS: 10.9g

NET CARBS: 9.6g

FIBER: 1.3g

PROTEIN: 43.4g

To make the spaghetti squash

1. Cut the spaghetti squash in half lengthwise and remove the seeds. Place each half facedown in a microwave-safe dish. Add the water. Microwave on high for 12 minutes.

2. Using a fork, scoop the squash from the shells.

3. In a large skillet over medium-high heat, heat 1 tablespoon of olive oil for about 1 minute. Add the squash to the skillet, stirring to allow any moisture to dissipate. Cook for about 7 minutes, until the squash begins to brown.

4. Remove it from the heat. Transfer the squash to a large bowl. Add ¼ cup of parsley to the bowl and set aside.

To make the meatballs

1. In a medium bowl, mix together the remaining ¼ cup of parsley, beef, pork, ¼ cup of Parmesan cheese, basil, oregano, onion powder, garlic, salt, and pepper.

2. Form the mixture into 12 meatballs.

3. In a large skillet over medium-high heat, heat the remaining tablespoon of oil olive for about 1 minute. Add the meatballs. Brown for 1 to 2 minutes on each side until fully browned, about 5 minutes total.

4. Add the pasta sauce to the pan. Stir to coat the meatballs thoroughly.

5. Reduce the heat to low. Cover the skillet. Cook for 10 to 15 minutes, or until the meatballs are cooked through.

6. Plate 3 meatballs and ¼ cup of sauce over one-quarter of the spaghetti squash per person. Sprinkle the remaining ¼ cup of Parmesan cheese evenly over the plated servings.

BARBECUE ONION AND GOAT CHEESE FLATBREAD

SERVES 2

PREP TIME: 20 MINUTES ▪ COOK TIME: 10 TO 15 MINUTES ▪ TOTAL TIME: 35 MINUTES

Flatbread is a lot like pizza crust except lighter and airier. This coconut flour-based flatbread is bubbly and crisp, perfect for the contrasting addition of barbecue sauce, onions, and goat cheese. If you have grilled chicken or other cooked meat on hand, add it to this dish for an extra dose of protein.

SNEAKY KETO CLASSICS

PER SERVING
(½ FLATBREAD PIZZA)

RATIO: 3:1
CALORIES: 565
TOTAL FAT: 38.7g
CARBS: 17.3g
NET CARBS: 13.3g
FIBER: 4g
PROTEIN: 35.7g

FOR THE FLATBREAD

2 tablespoons coconut flour

⅛ teaspoon baking powder

4 egg whites

¼ teaspoon onion powder

¼ teaspoon garlic powder

¼ cup coconut milk

FOR THE TOPPINGS

2 tablespoons sugar-free barbecue sauce

¾ cup goat cheese, crumbled

½ cup sliced yellow onion

½ teaspoon minced garlic

⅛ teaspoon freshly ground black pepper

To make the flatbread

1. In a medium bowl, whisk together the coconut flour, baking powder, egg whites, onion powder, garlic powder, and coconut milk until there are no lumps.

2. Heat a large skillet over medium-high heat. Pour the coconut batter into the skillet and rotate the pan so the batter coats the entire pan. Cook for 2 minutes, or until the edges brown. Flip. Cook for 1 to 2 minutes more.

3. Remove the flatbread from the pan.

To assemble the pizza

1. Preheat the oven to 425°F.

2. Top the cooked flatbread evenly with the barbecue sauce, goat cheese, onion, garlic, and pepper.

3. Place the flatbread on a baking sheet. Put it in the preheated oven. Bake for 5 to 7 minutes, or until the cheese melts.

4. Remove it from the oven. Cool the flatbread for 2 minutes before slicing and serving.

CLASSIC MOZZARELLA STICKS

SERVES 4

PREP TIME: 10 MINUTES ▪ COOK TIME: 15 MINUTES ▪ TOTAL TIME: 1½ HOURS

Almost straight from my childhood, these classic mozzarella sticks are just as good as the real breaded thing. A key ingredient here is the powdered Parmesan cheese. Since it is powdered, it mimics the adhesive qualities of breading, but without the carbs. Shredded Parmesan will not yield the same crispy exterior. When I've had a long day, I like to whip these up right when I come home, and then fry a batch for my favorite weeknight shows. These also freeze well if you prefer to make them in advance.

2 ounces powdered Parmesan cheese

1 teaspoon Italian seasoning

1 egg

5 mozzarella cheese sticks

Oil for frying

Pizza Sauce (page 225) or Ranch Dressing (page 218) for serving

PER SERVING (ABOUT 4 PIECES)

RATIO: 3:1

CALORIES: 275

TOTAL FAT: 22.1g

CARBS: 1.9g

NET CARBS: 1.9g

FIBER: 0g

PROTEIN: 21.1g

1. In a large bowl, combine the powdered Parmesan cheese and Italian seasoning.

2. In another bowl, whisk the egg for 1 minute.

3. On a cutting board, slice each mozzarella stick crosswise into thirds for 15 pieces total.

4. Dip one piece of the mozzarella into the egg and then roll it in the seasoned Parmesan cheese.

5. Re-dip the piece of cheese in the egg, and then again in the Parmesan cheese.

6. Roll the cheese-covered mozzarella piece between your hands so the coating adheres.

7. Repeat with remaining mozzarella pieces.

8. Freeze the cheese sticks for at least 1 hour.

9. When ready to cook, preheat 1 inch of oil in a large pan to 350°F.

(continued)

10. Place 2 to 3 cheese sticks in the pan at a time, being careful not to overcrowd. Cook for 4 to 6 minutes, turning halfway through.

11. Transfer to paper towels to drain.

12. Repeat with the remaining pieces.

13. Serve with Pizza Sauce (page 225) or Ranch Dressing (page 218).

SNEAKY KETO
CLASSICS

BAKED "SPAGHETTI"

SERVES 8
PREP TIME: 30 MINUTES ▪ COOK TIME: 1½ HOURS ▪ TOTAL TIME: 2 HOURS

Spaghetti is a staple of every family's weeknight meals. Enjoy this classic on keto by replacing the traditional noodles with spaghetti squash, which looks just like noodles when it's cooked. Topped with gobs of cheese and a hefty serving of sugar-free pasta sauce, this is a treat everyone will enjoy.

1 large spaghetti squash (yields 5 cups)

½ cup butter

½ pound 80-percent lean ground beef

½ pound Italian sausage

½ pound chicken sausage

½ cup red wine

1 large onion, diced

5 garlic cloves, minced

½ pound mushrooms, sliced

1 (6-ounce) can tomato paste

1 (18-ounce) can diced tomatoes

1 tablespoon Italian seasoning

4 ounces ricotta cheese, divided

4 ounces mozzarella cheese, divided

8 ounces grated Parmesan cheese, divided

½ teaspoon salt

½ teaspoon freshly ground black pepper

1. Preheat the oven to 350°F.

2. Place the spaghetti squash in a large microwaveable bowl and use the tip of a sharp knife to pierce the shell all around. Microwave on high for 15 to 20 minutes, depending on the size of your squash. Remove from the microwave. Set aside to cool.

3. Heat a large skillet over medium-high heat. Add the butter and melt for 1 to 2 minutes.

4. Add the ground beef, Italian sausage, and chicken sausage to the pan. Sauté for about 10 minutes.

5. Add the red wine and lower the heat to medium, letting the wine reduce with the meat for 3 to 5 minutes.

6. Add the onion and garlic. Cook until tender, about 4 minutes. Add the mushrooms and stir, cooking for an additional 8 to 9 minutes.

(continued)

7. Add the tomato paste, diced tomatoes with the juices, and Italian seasoning to the mixture. Stir well to combine. Cook for 10 to 15 minutes, until reduced by half.

8. Return to the spaghetti squash. Cut it in half lengthwise. Clean it, removing the inner seeds, and scoop out the flesh with a fork.

9. In a large baking dish with a lid, spread half of the spaghetti squash in the bottom. Top with 2 ounces of ricotta, 2 ounces of mozzarella, and 4 ounces of Parmesan. Cover with the tomato sauce. Top with the remaining half of the spaghetti squash.

10. Finish with the remaining 2 ounces of ricotta, 2 ounces of mozzarella, and 4 ounces of Parmesan cheese.

11. Cover the pan and put it in the preheated oven. Bake for 20 minutes.

12. Remove the dish from the oven and carefully remove the lid. Return the uncovered dish to the oven and bake for another 15 to 20 minutes. Finish with 2 to 3 minutes under the broiler for a crispy, browned top.

13. Cool for 10 to 15 minutes before serving.

SNEAKY KETO
CLASSICS

TOFU FRIES

SERVES 2

PREP TIME: 15 MINUTES · COOK TIME: 15 MINUTES · TOTAL TIME: 30 MINUTES

If you're missing fries with that burger and shake, don't despair—try this recipe for tofu fries with a crispy-on-the-outside and moist-on-the-inside texture. Paired with Sugar-Free Ketchup (page 216) or garlic aioli, it's hard to tell these from the real deal. Make sure to remove as much moisture as possible before frying for the crispiest texture.

Oil for frying

1 package (12 ounces) extra-firm tofu, sliced into ¼-inch slices

1 tablespoon salt

2 teaspoons freshly ground black pepper

1 teaspoon ground cumin

1 teaspoon dried parsley

1 teaspoon garlic powder

½ teaspoon onion powder

¼ teaspoon paprika

¼ teaspoon cayenne pepper

Sugar-Free Ketchup (page 216) for serving

SNEAKY KETO CLASSICS

PER SERVING (6 OUNCES TOFU FRIES)

RATIO: 3:1

CALORIES: 197

TOTAL FAT: 14.3g

CARBS: 6.5g

NET CARBS: 4g

FIBER: 2.5g

PROTEIN: 14.7g

1. In a large pot, heat about 4 inches of oil to 350°F.

2. Dry each tofu slice thoroughly between paper towels or a dishcloth.

3. In a medium bowl, mix together the salt, black pepper, cumin, parsley, garlic powder, onion powder, paprika, and cayenne pepper.

4. Dredge the tofu fries in the spice mixture and set aside.

5. Working in batches, add a few fries at a time to the oil so they do not stick together. Cook each batch for about 4 minutes, or until golden brown. Remove from the oil with a slotted spoon. Set aside on paper towels to drain.

6. Repeat the process with the remaining tofu strips, working in batches as needed.

7. Serve with Sugar-Free Ketchup (page 216).

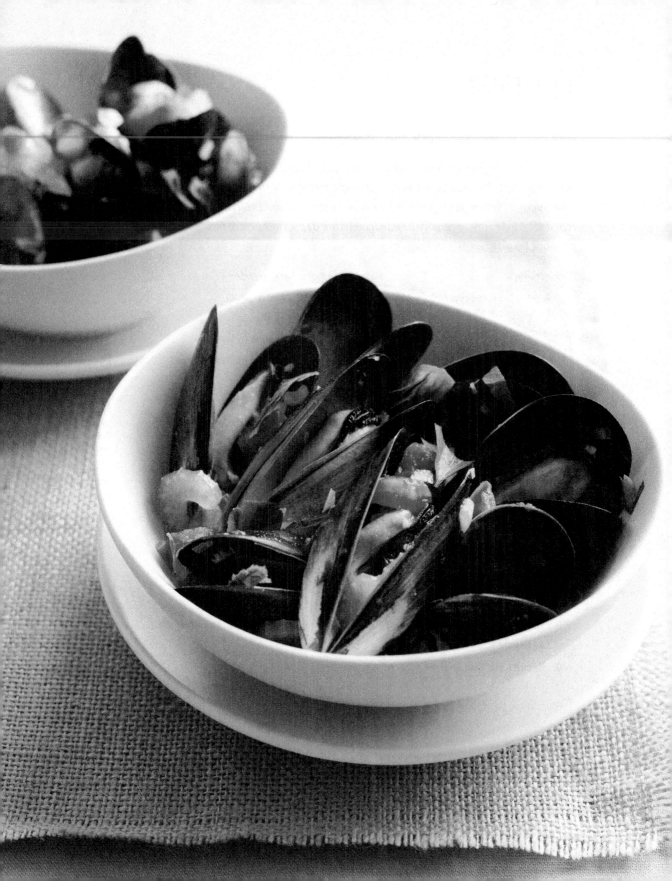

CHAPTER
6

FISHY
FAVORITES

STEAMED MUSSELS WITH GARLIC AND THYME

SERVES 8

PREP TIME: 25 MINUTES ▪ COOK TIME: 20 MINUTES ▪ TOTAL TIME: 45 MINUTES

While freshly steamed mussels are higher in carbohydrate than many other shellfish, nothing beats the taste. Paired with fresh thyme and a heaping serving of garlic, these flavorful morsels are perfect for an appetizer or a main course. Serve with toasted Coconut Almond Flour Bread (page 105) or a crunchy vegetable medley, like celery and bell peppers.

4 pounds live mussels, cleaned, scrubbed, and debearded

½ cup butter

3 tablespoons olive oil

½ cup diced onion

4 garlic cloves, minced

½ cup diced tomato

1 tablespoon fresh thyme

½ cup white wine

1 cup chicken or seafood broth

2 tablespoons freshly squeezed lemon juice

½ teaspoon salt

¼ teaspoon freshly ground black pepper

PER SERVING

RATIO: 3:1

CALORIES: 374

TOTAL FAT: 22.5g

CARBS: 11.5g

NET CARBS: 11.1g

FIBER: 0.4g

PROTEIN: 28.4g

1. Place the cleaned mussels in a large bowl. Cover with cool water. Set aside.

2. In a large, heavy pot over medium heat, heat the butter and olive oil for about 1 minute. Add the onions. Cook for 3 to 5 minutes, until translucent. Add the garlic and cook for 1 to 2 minutes more.

3. Add the tomato, thyme, white wine, broth, lemon juice, salt, and pepper. Increase the heat and bring the mixture to a boil.

4. Add the mussels and cover the pot. Cook for 8 to 10 minutes, shaking the pot at various intervals to allow the mussels to cook evenly.

5. Pour the steaming mussels into a bowl. Discard any that are unopened. Serve immediately.

COCONUT SHRIMP

SERVES 6

PREP TIME: 15 MINUTES ▪ COOK TIME: 15 MINUTES ▪ TOTAL TIME: 30 MINUTES

Nothing says tropical paradise like a batch of coconut shrimp. Paired with a tangy aioli, these are just as good as the non-keto version, if not better.

FOR THE COCONUT SHRIMP

Oil for frying

1 cup unsweetened shredded coconut

½ cup unsweetened flaked coconut

¼ cup unsweetened coconut milk

½ cup mayonnaise

2 egg yolks

¼ teaspoon salt

⅛ teaspoon freshly ground black pepper

½ teaspoon garlic powder

1 pound shrimp, peeled and deveined, tails left on

FOR THE AIOLI

½ cup mayonnaise

2 tablespoons chili sauce, such as Huy Fong Foods brand

2 teaspoons freshly squeezed lime juice

1 teaspoon red pepper flakes

PER SERVING

RATIO: 4:1

CALORIES: 466

TOTAL FAT: 40.8g

CARBS: 6g

NET CARBS: 3.8g

FIBER: 2.2g

PROTEIN: 19.2g

To make the coconut shrimp

1. In a large pot, heat 2 inches of oil to 350°F for deep-frying.

2. In a medium bowl, thoroughly mix together the shredded coconut, flaked coconut, coconut milk, mayonnaise, egg yolks, salt, pepper, and garlic powder.

3. Using 1 to 2 tablespoons of batter, carefully form it around each shrimp, leaving the tails exposed.

4. Immediately drop the battered shrimp into the preheated oil. Repeat with 2 to 3 more shrimp. Cook for 4 to 6 minutes, until golden brown.

5. Remove the shrimp from the oil. Set aside to cool on a paper-towel-lined plate. Repeat the process with the remaining shrimp.

To make the aioli

1. In a small bowl, thoroughly combine the mayonnaise, chili sauce, lime juice, and red pepper flakes.

2. Serve immediately with the coconut shrimp.

GRILLED SHRIMP WITH AVOCADO SALAD

SERVES 3

PREP TIME: 20 MINUTES ▪ COOK TIME: 5 MINUTES ▪ TOTAL TIME: 25 MINUTES

This light but refreshing combination of grilled shrimp and avocado gets its inspiration from traditional dishes served on tropical islands. Remember, shrimp cook quickly and can be overcooked easily. Avocados are also delicate, and should be handled minimally before serving.

1 pound shrimp, peeled and deveined

2 tablespoons olive oil

½ teaspoon garlic powder

½ teaspoon salt, divided

⅛ teaspoon freshly ground black pepper

1 avocado, peeled, pitted, and diced

¼ cup chopped bell pepper

¼ cup chopped tomato

¼ cup chopped onion

1 teaspoon freshly squeezed lime juice

FISHY FAVORITES

PER SERVING

RATIO: 3:1

CALORIES: 409

TOTAL FAT: 25g

CARBS: 10.9g

NET CARBS: 5.8g

FIBER: 5.1g

PROTEIN: 36.1g

1. Heat a griddle over medium-high heat.

2. In a large bowl, combine the shrimp, olive oil, garlic powder, ¼ teaspoon of salt, and pepper. Mix until the shrimp are coated thoroughly.

3. In a medium bowl, mix together the avocado, bell pepper, tomato, onion, and lime juice. Sprinkle with the remaining ¼ teaspoon of salt. Set aside in the refrigerator.

4. Place the shrimp on the hot griddle, on their sides. Cook for 2 to 3 minutes. Flip, and cook for another 1 to 2 minutes. Remove the shrimp from the griddle.

5. Plate with the avocado salad to serve.

SHRIMP SCAMPI WITH ZUCCHINI NOODLES

SERVES 3
PREP TIME: 20 MINUTES · COOK TIME: 10 MINUTES · TOTAL TIME: 30 MINUTES

Shrimp scampi is a pasta classic that gets a twist in this "keto-fied" recipe by substituting zucchini noodles for the pasta. A spiralizer, used to create the zucchini noodles for this dish, is a versatile tool to invest in for your kitchen arsenal that is extremely useful on the keto diet. If you have a mandolin, you can also achieve the unique "zoodles" cut with that.

2 tablespoons olive oil

1 tablespoon minced garlic

1 pound shrimp, peeled and deveined

¼ cup dry white wine

2 tablespoons freshly squeezed lemon juice

1 tablespoon butter

3 tablespoons heavy (whipping) cream

2½ cups zucchini noodles

¼ teaspoon salt

¼ teaspoon freshly ground black pepper

1 tablespoon chopped fresh parsley

PER SERVING
RATIO: 3:1
CALORIES: 384
TOTAL FAT: 21.6g
CARBS: 7.7g
NET CARBS: 6.5g
FIBER: 1.2g
PROTEIN: 36.3g

1. Heat a large skillet over medium heat. Add the olive oil and heat for about 1 minute. Add the garlic. Cook for 1 minute.

2. Add the shrimp to the pan. Cook on all sides, turning, about 4 minutes. Remove the shrimp from the pan. Set aside, leaving the liquid in the pan.

3. To the pan with the reserved liquid, add the white wine and lemon juice. Scrape the bottom of the pan to incorporate any solids with the liquid, stirring constantly for 2 minutes.

4. Add the butter and heavy cream. Cook for 1 minute.

5. Add the zucchini noodles to the pan. Cook, stirring occasionally, for about 2 minutes or until the zucchini is al dente (noodle-like) in texture.

6. Return the shrimp to the pan. Season with the salt and pepper. Stir to incorporate all ingredients.

7. Plate and garnish with fresh parsley. Serve immediately.

CILANTRO LIME SHRIMP AND VEGETABLE KEBABS WITH CHIPOTLE SOUR CREAM SAUCE

SERVES 2

PREP TIME: 20 MINUTES · COOK TIME: 10 MINUTES · TOTAL TIME: 30 MINUTES

For a Mexican-flavored kick, try these cilantro and lime shrimp kebabs. With their layers of onion and bell pepper, these delicious kebabs can be made indoors or out (though they benefit, of course, from the smokiness of a grill). If you are unable to use a grill, you can add ½ teaspoon of liquid smoke to the shrimp marinade.

PER SERVING
RATIO: 3:1
CALORIES: 410
TOTAL FAT: 23g
CARBS: 9.9g
NET CARBS: 8.7g
FIBER: 1.2g
PROTEIN: 40.3g

FOR THE SHRIMP

¾ pound shrimp, peeled and deveined

2 tablespoons olive oil

2 tablespoons freshly squeezed lime juice

½ teaspoon garlic powder, divided

½ teaspoon onion powder, divided

¼ cup chopped fresh cilantro

¼ teaspoon salt

¼ teaspoon freshly ground black pepper

½ teaspoon liquid smoke (optional)

½ cup roughly chopped bell pepper

⅓ cup roughly chopped onion

FOR THE CHIPOTLE SOUR CREAM SAUCE

¼ cup sour cream

1 teaspoon chipotle pepper powder

To make the shrimp

1. Heat a grill, or griddle, to medium-high heat.

2. In a large bowl, combine the shrimp, olive oil, lime juice, ¼ teaspoon garlic powder, ¼ teaspoon onion powder, cilantro, salt, and pepper. If cooking indoors, add the liquid smoke (if using).

3. Mix until the shrimp are coated thoroughly.

To make the chipotle sour cream sauce

In a small bowl, mix the sour cream, chipotle powder, the remaining ¼ teaspoon garlic powder, and the remaining ¼ teaspoon onion powder. Refrigerate until ready to serve.

To make the kebabs

1. Skewer the shrimp, alternating with the bell peppers and onions.

2. Place the kebabs on the preheated grill. Cook for 3 to 5 minutes. Flip, and cook for 3 to 5 minutes more.

3. Remove from the grill. Check the shrimp for doneness. The shrimp is done when firm in texture, opaque, and tinged with its signature pink-orange color.

4. Remove the shrimp and vegetables from the kebabs. Serve with the chipotle sour cream sauce.

FISHY
FAVORITES

SHRIMP, BAMBOO SHOOT, AND BROCCOLI STIR-FRY

SERVES 2

PREP TIME: 15 MINUTES ▪ COOK TIME: 15 MINUTES ▪ TOTAL TIME: 30 MINUTES

Chinese food may seem like a world away while eating on the keto diet, but not with this modified stir-fry. Pair this with Cauliflower "Rice" (page 98) or enjoy on its own. It is equally good both ways. The bamboo shoots provide a nice texture alongside the shrimp and broccoli for a filling meal.

2 tablespoons olive oil

¾ pound shrimp, peeled and deveined

1 tablespoon minced garlic

1 cup sliced bamboo shoots

¼ cup chopped onion

1 cup broccoli florets

½ teaspoon sesame oil

3 tablespoons soy sauce

½ teaspoon unsweetened rice wine vinegar

½ teaspoon Chinese five-spice powder

¼ teaspoon freshly ground black pepper

PER SERVING

RATIO: 3:1

CALORIES: 394

TOTAL FAT: 18.4g

CARBS: 14.2g

NET CARBS: 107g

FIBER: 3.5g

PROTEIN: 43.9

1. Heat a large skillet over medium-high heat. Add the olive oil and heat for 1 minute.

2. Add the shrimp and garlic to the skillet. Cook for 2 to 3 minutes, or until the shrimp are mostly cooked. Remove the shrimp from the skillet.

3. Lower the heat to medium. Add the bamboo shoots, onion, and broccoli and sauté for 5 to 8 minutes, or until room temperature. Add the sesame oil, soy sauce, rice wine vinegar, Chinese five-spice powder, and black pepper. Mix to combine.

4. Add the shrimp back to the skillet, and cook for another 1 to 2 minutes.

5. Serve immediately.

BACON-WRAPPED SCALLOPS AND BROCCOLINI

SERVES 3

PREP TIME: 15 MINUTES ▪ COOK TIME: 15 MINUTES ▪ TOTAL TIME: 30 MINUTES

Scallops are delicate seafood that can take on many flavors easily. In this recipe, they take on the rich flavor of bacon alongside a buttery serving of broccolini. If you have not tried broccolini, it is very similar to other cruciferous vegetables. A cross between broccoli and kai-lan, it is high in fiber and packed full of vitamin C.

5 bacon slices

1 pound scallops (about 10)

½ teaspoon salt, divided

¼ teaspoon freshly ground black pepper, divided

4 tablespoons (½ stick) butter, divided

15 broccolini pieces

1 teaspoon minced garlic

2 tablespoons dry white wine

2 teaspoons olive oil

PER SERVING
(3 BACON-WRAPPED
SCALLOPS)

RATIO: 3:1

CALORIES: 510

TOTAL FAT: 35.4g

CARBS: 8.7g

NET CARBS: 7.9g

FIBER: 0.8g

PROTEIN: 41.5g

1. Cut the bacon slices in half crosswise, creating 10 small slices. Wrap one slice around each scallop, securing with a toothpick. Season with ¼ teaspoon of salt and ⅛ teaspoon of pepper.

2. Heat a medium skillet over medium-high heat. Add 3 tablespoons of butter and heat for 2 minutes.

3. Add the broccolini, garlic, and wine. Sauté for 2 minutes. Cover and reduce the heat to medium-low.

4. Heat a large skillet over medium-high heat. Add the remaining tablespoon of butter and the olive oil and heat for 2 minutes.

5. Increase the heat under the large skillet to high. Add the scallops. Sear for 1½ minutes per side. Roll the scallops onto their sides so the bacon crisps. Cook for about 1 minute on each side.

6. Check the broccolini for doneness. Season with the remaining ¼ teaspoon of salt and ⅛ teaspoon of pepper.

7. Plate immediately with the scallops, saucing with any excess garlic butter from the pan.

FRUGAL FRIENDLY TIP: Frozen scallops are usually a few dollars cheaper per pound and still fresh, as most are flash-frozen as soon as they are caught.

CRAB CAKES WITH GARLIC AIOLI

SERVES 4

PREP TIME: 15 MINUTES • COOK TIME: 15 MINUTES • TOTAL TIME: 30 MINUTES

Few things in life make me as happy as crab cakes. Usually crab cakes are breaded or utilize breadcrumbs to hold them together, but this favorite recipe of mine uses Parmesan cheese and coconut flour to bind the meat. Crispy and flavorful, I can't get enough of these and will often double the recipe, freezing some for a lazy night when I don't feel like working hard on dinner. Remember when buying crabmeat that it is machine separated, so always check for shells before using.

PER SERVING
RATIO: 3:1
CALORIES: 576
FAT: 46.4g
CARBS: 10.5g
NET CARBS: 7.4g
FIBER: 3.1g
PROTEIN: 31.9g

FOR THE CRAB CAKES

½ pound jumbo lump crabmeat

½ pound lump crabmeat

¼ cup mayonnaise

1 egg, beaten

¼ cup coconut flour

1 teaspoon mustard

1 teaspoon seafood seasoning

¼ teaspoon paprika

1 teaspoon minced garlic

¼ cup finely chopped onion

¼ cup finely chopped bell pepper

1 tablespoon finely chopped fresh parsley

¼ teaspoon salt

¼ teaspoon freshly ground black pepper

1 cup shredded Parmesan cheese

3 tablespoons butter

FOR THE AIOLI

2 teaspoons minced garlic

1 tablespoon freshly squeezed lemon juice

1 egg

½ teaspoon salt

⅛ teaspoon freshly ground black pepper

½ cup olive oil

To make the crab cakes

1. In a large bowl, combine the jumbo lump crabmeat, lump crabmeat, mayonnaise, egg, coconut flour, mustard, seafood seasoning, paprika, garlic, onion, bell pepper, parsley, salt, and pepper. Mix well.

2. Mix in the Parmesan cheese. Divide the crabmeat mixture into six equal portions. Form each into a patty. Refrigerate to firm up while making the aioli.

To make the aioli

1. In a food processor, mix the garlic and lemon juice until smooth.

2. Add the egg, salt, and pepper. Purée, while slowly adding the olive oil until the aioli forms. Set aside.

To finish the dish

1. Heat a large skillet over medium-high heat. Add the butter. Cook for 1 minute.

2. Gently add the crab cakes to the pan. Cook for 7 minutes, being careful not to burn the butter. Reduce the heat to medium. Flip the cakes. Cook for 5 to 7 minutes more, or until done. Transfer the crab cakes to paper towels to drain.

3. Serve immediately with half of the aioli. Refrigerate the remaining aioli stored in an airtight container.

FISHY
FAVORITES

PARMESAN-CRUSTED TILAPIA WITH SAUTÉED SPINACH

SERVES 2

PREP TIME: 15 MINUTES ▪ COOK TIME: 15 MINUTES ▪ TOTAL TIME: 30 MINUTES

Parmesan is an excellent crusting cheese that can substitute for bread crumbs in many recipes. For this tilapia, the Parmesan gets an added boost from almond flour, allowing it to bind to the fish more easily and stay put while it cooks. With a side of sautéed spinach, this is a heart-healthy meal that's great for any weeknight.

½ cup grated Parmesan cheese

2 tablespoons almond flour

1 teaspoon paprika

¼ teaspoon salt

⅛ teaspoon freshly ground black pepper

2 tilapia fillets

2 tablespoons olive oil, divided

1½ cups spinach

½ teaspoon garlic powder

1 tablespoon chopped fresh parsley

PER SERVING
(1 TILAPIA FILLET,
½ OF THE SPINACH)

RATIO: 3:1

CALORIES: 376

TOTAL FAT: 26.6g

CARBS: 4.1g

NET CARBS: 2.4g

FIBER: 1.7g

PROTEIN: 32g

1. Preheat the oven to 400°F.

2. In a medium bowl, mix together the Parmesan cheese, almond flour, paprika, salt, and pepper.

3. Place the tilapia fillets on a plate and drizzle with 1 tablespoon of olive oil. Massage the oil into the fish, and then dredge them in the Parmesan mix, coating thoroughly.

4. Line a baking dish with aluminum foil. Place the fillets inside. Put the dish in the preheated oven and bake for 10 to 15 minutes, depending on the thickness of the fillets.

5. While the fillets cook, add the remaining tablespoon of olive oil to a large skillet and heat over medium-high heat.

6. Add the spinach and sauté until tender, about 6 minutes.

7. Add the garlic powder. Cover, and reduce the heat to medium-low. Cook for 3 to 5 minutes.

8. Remove the baking dish from the oven. Check the fillets for doneness.

9. Plate the spinach with the fillets on top and serve immediately, garnished with the parsley.

SESAME GINGER SALMON WITH CAULIFLOWER MASH

SERVES 2

PREP TIME: 20 MINUTES ▪ COOK TIME: 20 MINUTES ▪ TOTAL TIME: 40 MINUTES

Nutty sesame pairs with bright ginger in this Asian-inspired salmon recipe served with Cauliflower Mash (page 99). Leftovers of this great weekday meal can be reheated easily for lunch the next day. If you want to enjoy these "mashed potatoes" with another meal, double the amount of ingredients and save half for later—they freeze well.

1 tablespoon minced fresh ginger

½ teaspoon sesame oil

1 teaspoon olive oil

½ teaspoon rice wine vinegar

1 teaspoon soy sauce

2 (8-ounce) salmon fillets

FISHY FAVORITES

PER SERVING
(1 SALMON FILLET)

RATIO: 3:1

CALORIES: 539

TOTAL FAT: 39.5g

CARBS: 7.3g

NET CARBS: 5g

FIBER: 2.3g

PROTEIN: 41.8g

1. Preheat the oven to 400°F.

2. In a medium bowl, mix together the ginger, sesame oil, olive oil, rice vinegar, and soy sauce.

3. Add the salmon fillets. Cover completely with the sauce.

4. Line a baking dish with aluminum foil. Place the fillets inside. Pour any remaining sauce over the fillets.

5. Put the dish into the preheated oven. Bake for 15 to 20 minutes, depending on the thickness of the fillets.

6. Remove the dish from the oven and check the fillets for doneness.

7. Serve immediately with the Cauliflower Mash (page 99).

CHARRED ALASKAN SALMON WITH GARLIC GREEN BEANS

SERVES 4
PREP TIME: 15 MINUTES ▪ COOK TIME: 25 MINUTES ▪ TOTAL TIME: 40 MINUTES

Salmon is a perennial favorite at most dinner tables, but some people (like my significant other) can't get past the specific flavor of salmon. For those folks (and my live-in taste tester), try this recipe, which is bursting with spices and accompanied by my favorite side dish, garlicky green beans. Allow the salmon to marinate in the rub overnight for the best flavor.

PER SERVING
(1 SALMON FILLET)
RATIO: 3:1
CALORIES: 539
TOTAL FAT: 42.2g
CARBS: 12.3g
NET CARBS: 6.6g
FIBER: 5.7g
PROTEIN: 31.3g

FOR THE RUB

2 tablespoons stevia, or other sugar substitute

1 tablespoon chili powder

1 teaspoon freshly ground black pepper

½ tablespoon ground cumin

½ tablespoon paprika

½ tablespoon salt

¼ teaspoon dry mustard

Dash cinnamon

FOR THE SALMON

4 tablespoons coconut oil

4 (4- to 6-ounce) Alaskan salmon fillets

4 tablespoons Dijon mustard, divided

FOR THE GREEN BEANS

3 tablespoons butter

1 tablespoon olive oil

4 garlic cloves, minced

1 pound green beans

½ teaspoon salt

¼ teaspoon freshly ground black pepper

To make the rub

In a medium bowl, combine the stevia, chili powder, black pepper, cumin, paprika, salt, dry mustard, and cinnamon.

To prepare the salmon

1. In a large skillet over medium heat, heat the coconut oil for about 5 minutes.

2. Liberally coat each salmon fillet with 1 tablespoon of mustard.

3. Season each fillet, on both sides, with an equal amount of the rub. Set aside.

4. Once the coconut oil has heated, increase the heat to medium-high. Add the salmon and sear for about 2 minutes. Flip and reduce the heat to medium. Cook for 6 to 8 minutes more, until the fish is opaque.

To make the green beans

1. In another large skillet over medium heat, heat the butter and olive oil. Add the garlic and cook until fragrant, about 1 minute.

2. Add the green beans, salt, and pepper. Cover and reduce the heat to medium-low. Cook for 10 to 12 minutes, stirring occasionally.

3. Serve immediately alongside the salmon.

INGREDIENT TIP: If Alaskan salmon is not available, feel free to substitute any other type of fresh salmon.

TERIYAKI SALMON WITH SPICY MAYO AND ASPARAGUS

SERVES 2

PREP TIME: 20 MINUTES ▪ COOK TIME: 25 MINUTES ▪ TOTAL TIME: 45 MINUTES

While teriyaki sauce traditionally does contain sugar, our keto-friendly version on page 215 uses a sugar-free substitute that is still highly comparable and tastes almost the same on a protein like salmon, which absorbs flavors very well. Topped with a spicy aioli, this flaky fish dish is served with buttered asparagus for a classic-style dinner. If you enjoy an added crunch, toss some slivered almonds in with the asparagus right before serving.

PER SERVING
(1 SALMON FILLET,
6 ASPARAGUS)
RATIO: 3:1
CALORIES: 577
TOTAL FAT: 42.2g
CARBS: 12.9g
NET CARBS: 9.6g
FIBER: 3.3g
PROTEIN: 41.5g

FOR THE SPICY MAYO

2 teaspoons minced garlic

1 tablespoon freshly squeezed lemon juice

1 egg

½ teaspoon salt

1 tablespoon cayenne pepper

⅛ teaspoon freshly ground black pepper

½ cup olive oil

FOR SALMON AND ASPARAGUS

12 asparagus spears

½ teaspoon minced fresh ginger

2 teaspoons olive oil, divided

½ teaspoon rice wine vinegar

¼ teaspoon freshly ground black pepper

4 tablespoons Teriyaki Sauce (page 215), or purchased sugar-free teriyaki sauce (such as Seal Sama)

2 (8-ounce) salmon fillets

Sliced scallions, for garnish

To make the spicy mayo

1. In a food processor, mix the garlic and lemon juice until smooth.

2. Add the egg, salt, cayenne pepper, and black pepper to the garlic and lemon juice purée. While puréeing, slowly add the olive oil until the mayo forms. Set aside in the refrigerator while the fillets cook.

To make the salmon and asparagus

1. Preheat the oven to 400°F.

2. Remove the woody ends from the asparagus, leaving only the tender portion of the stalk.

3. In a medium bowl, mix together the ginger, 1 teaspoon of olive oil, rice wine vinegar, pepper, and the Teriyaki Sauce (page 215).

4. Add the salmon and cover completely with the sauce.

5. Line a baking dish with aluminum foil. Transfer the salmon from the sauce to the dish. Pour any remaining sauce over the fillets. Tuck the asparagus around the fillets and drizzle them with the remaining teaspoon of olive oil.

6. Put the dish in the preheated oven. Bake for 15 to 20 minutes, depending on the thickness of the fillets.

7. Remove the dish from the oven and check the fillets for doneness.

8. Serve immediately with half of the spicy mayo. Garnish with the scallions. Refrigerate the remaining mayo in an airtight container.

SMOKED SALMON AVOCADO SUSHI ROLL

SERVES 4

PREP TIME: 15 MINUTES · COOK TIME: 20 MINUTES · TOTAL TIME: 35 MINUTES

Sushi cravings while on the keto diet are a real challenge. While sashimi is still fair game, getting the experience of a sushi roll without rice is often difficult at most restaurants. Make your own with this simple recipe that has all the flavors of your favorite sushi. Serve with pickled ginger and low-carb soy sauce.

14 ounces smoked salmon

1 tablespoon wasabi paste (optional)

¾ cup cream cheese, at room temperature

½ avocado, sliced

1 tablespoon sesame seeds

FISHY
FAVORITES

PER SERVING
RATIO: 3:1
CALORIES: 539
TOTAL FAT: 42.2g
CARBS: 12.3g
NET CARBS: 6.6g
FIBER: 5.7g
PROTEIN: 31.3g

1. On a cutting board, lay out a large piece of plastic wrap.

2. Place the salmon pieces on the plastic wrap, overlapping, to create a large rectangle 6 to 7 inches long and 4 inches wide.

3. In a small bowl, mix together the wasabi paste (if using) and the cream cheese.

4. Spread the cream cheese evenly over the entire smoked salmon rectangle.

5. Arrange the avocado over the cream cheese, in the center of the rectangle.

6. Grabbing the plastic wrap at one end, lift and carefully begin to roll the salmon. Hold the plastic wrap tightly over the roll as you go to apply pressure to hold it together.

7. Unwrap the plastic wrap from the sushi roll.

8. Cover the sushi roll in sesame seeds, patting them into the outer layer.

9. Refrigerate the roll for 15 to 20 minutes.

10. With a very sharp knife, slice into pieces and serve.

ROASTED COD WITH GARLIC BUTTER AND BOK CHOY

SERVES 2

PREP TIME: 5 MINUTES • COOK TIME: 20 MINUTES • TOTAL TIME: 25 MINUTES

This recipe for roasted cod with bok choy is a personal favorite. Quick to make with the aluminum-foil steaming method, this dish will impress with little effort. Bok choy is available year-round, but its peak season is winter. If you're making this dish during other times of the year, substitute a more seasonal vegetable, like broccoli or broccoli raab.

2 (8-ounce) cod fillets

¼ cup (½ stick) butter, thinly sliced

1 tablespoon minced garlic

½ pound baby bok choy, halved lengthwise

¼ teaspoon salt

¼ teaspoon freshly ground black pepper

PER SERVING
(1 COD FILLET, ½ OF
THE BOK CHOY)

RATIO: 3:1

CALORIES: 317

TOTAL FAT: 23.8g

CARBS: 4g

NET CARBS: 2.7g

FIBER: 1.3g

PROTEIN: 22.6g

1. Preheat the oven to 400°F.

2. Make a large pouch from aluminum foil and place the cod inside. Top with slices of butter and the garlic, evenly divided.

3. Tuck the bok choy around the fillets. Season with the salt and pepper.

4. Close the pouch with the two ends of the foil meeting at the top, so the butter remains in the pouch.

5. Place the sealed pouches in a baking dish. Put the dish in the preheated oven, and bake for 15 to 20 minutes, depending on the thickness of the fillets.

6. Remove the dish from the oven and check the fillets for doneness.

7. Serve immediately.

ROASTED TROUT WITH SWISS CHARD

SERVES 4

PREP TIME: 30 MINUTES · COOK TIME: 15 MINUTES · TOTAL TIME: 45 MINUTES

After a long day out fishing, nothing tastes better than a simply roasted trout and some fresh vegetables. Even if the catch came from the supermarket, trout is an incredibly delicious fish and cooks very easily with this recipe's foil method. Paired with fresh dill and fennel, the fish is impressive in flavor and presentation.

1 teaspoon salt, divided

½ teaspoon freshly ground black pepper, divided

4 (8-ounce) trout, cleaned

4 fresh dill sprigs

4 fresh fennel sprigs

2 pounds Swiss chard, cleaned and leaves separated from stems

4 tablespoons olive oil, divided

4 tablespoons butter, divided

1 lemon, quartered

4 tablespoons dry vermouth, or white wine, divided

PER SERVING (1 TROUT, ¼ SWISS CHARD)

RATIO: 3:1

CALORIES: 556

TOTAL FAT: 36.1g

CARBS: 11.4g

NET CARBS: 7g

FIBER: 4.4g

PROTEIN: 43.6g

1. Preheat the oven to 450°F.

2. Using ½ teaspoon of salt and ¼ teaspoon of pepper, season the insides of the trout. Place 1 dill sprig and 1 fennel sprig inside each trout.

3. Cut the Swiss chard stems into 2-inch pieces. Cut the leaves crosswise into 1½-inch strips. Set aside.

4. Cut four large pieces of aluminum foil into oval shapes large enough to fit one trout and one-quarter of the Swiss chard, with room enough to be sealed.

5. Using ¾ tablespoon of olive oil, brush the trout. Place one trout in the center of each piece of foil. Top each trout with one-quarter of the Swiss chard.

6. Season the trout with the remaining ½ teaspoon of salt, ¼ teaspoon of pepper, and 3¼ tablespoons of olive oil. Top each trout with 1 tablespoon of butter.

7. Squeeze a lemon quarter over each Swiss chard and trout bundle. Spoon 1 tablespoon of vermouth over each, as well. Close and seal the foil pouches tightly.

8. Place the foil packets on a baking sheet. Bake in the preheated oven for 10 to 12 minutes, depending on the thickness of the fish.

9. Remove from the oven and allow the packets to cool for 1 to 2 minutes before opening. Serve in the foil packet.

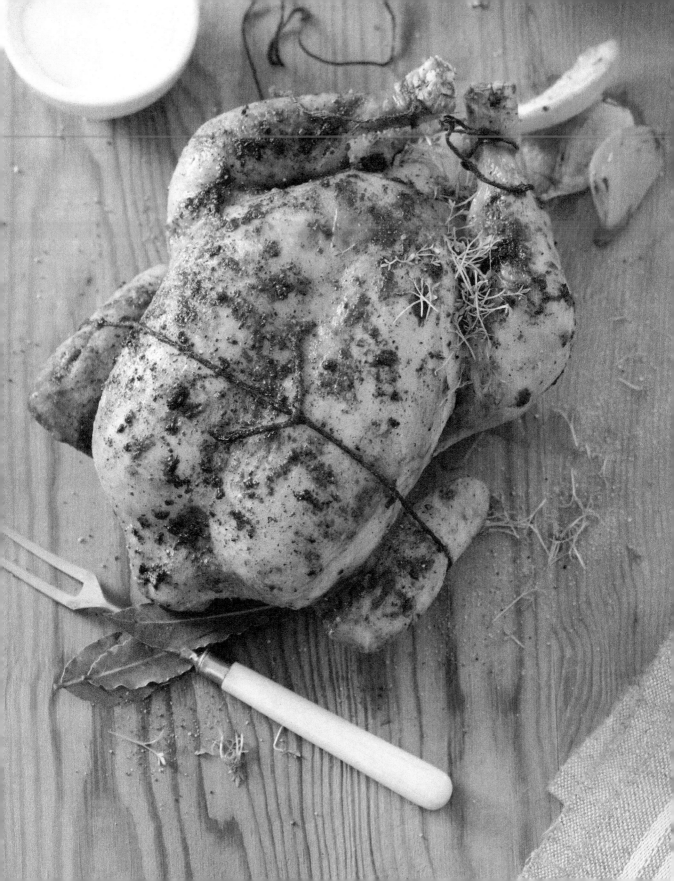

CHAPTER
7

PERFECT POULTRY

MUSTARD SHALLOT CHICKEN DRUMSTICKS

SERVES 4

PREP TIME: 15 MINUTES — COOK TIME: 20 MINUTES — TOTAL TIME: 35 MINUTES

Tangy and flavorful, these drumsticks are smothered in mustard, shallots, and white wine for a simple preparation. The fresh herbs and cream sauce pair well with a steamed vegetable, like broccoli, topped with butter. In some dishes, shallots can substitute for a combination of garlic and onion. The unique flavor of the shallot is important for this dish, so shallots should be used, if possible.

1½ pounds chicken drumsticks

¼ teaspoon salt

¼ teaspoon freshly ground black pepper

2 tablespoons butter

3 tablespoons finely chopped shallots

2 fresh thyme sprigs

1 tablespoon balsamic vinegar

¼ cup dry white wine

1 teaspoon Worcestershire sauce

½ cup chicken broth

2 teaspoons tomato paste

½ cup heavy (whipping) cream

1 tablespoon Dijon mustard

2 tablespoons finely chopped fresh parsley

1. Season the drumsticks with the salt and pepper. Set aside.

2. In a large skillet over medium-high heat, melt the butter. Add the drumsticks, skin-side down. Cook for 6 to 7 minutes, until browned. Turn the drumsticks on their sides. Cook for 2 minutes more. Turn the drumsticks again to the remaining uncooked side. Cook for 3 to 4 minutes more. With a meat thermometer, check the internal temperature. The chicken should reach 165°F before it is removed from the skillet.

3. Transfer the cooked chicken to a serving dish. Keep warm.

4. To any butter remaining in the skillet, add the shallots and thyme. Cook for 1 minute, until the shallots are tender.

5. Add the vinegar, white wine, and Worcestershire sauce. Bring the mixture to a boil.

6. Stir in the chicken broth. Return the mixture to a boil.

7. Add the tomato paste. Stir to combine. Cook for 5 to 6 minutes, or until the mixture reduces by half.

8. Once reduced, add the heavy cream. Bring to a boil again. Whisk in the mustard. You will have about 1 cup of sauce.

9. Pour the sauce over the drumsticks. Allow the drumsticks to rest for 2 minutes.

10. Garnish with the chopped parsley, and serve.

HERB ROASTED WHOLE CHICKEN WITH JICAMA

SERVES 4

PREP TIME: 15 MINUTES · COOK TIME: 1¼ HOURS · TOTAL TIME: 1¾ HOURS

A kitchen classic, roasted chicken is great not only for a family meal but also for leftovers—you can slice chicken breast for sandwiches or wraps, and chop up the meat for things like chicken salad. The basic herb blend in this recipe can be changed to whatever rubs you like to use. Jicama, full of fiber, roasts well with the chicken for a texture similar to roasted potatoes.

1 shallot, minced

2 fresh thyme sprigs, chopped

2 fresh rosemary sprigs, chopped

2 garlic cloves, minced

2 fresh sage sprigs, chopped

2 tablespoons chopped fresh parsley

1 (5-pound) whole roasting chicken

¼ cup olive oil

1 cup roughly chopped jicama

½ teaspoon salt

¼ teaspoon freshly ground black pepper

PER SERVING

RATIO: 3:1

CALORIES: 604

TOTAL FAT: 48.8g

CARBS: 3.4g

NET CARBS: 1.8g

FIBER: 1.6g

PROTEIN: 38.5g

1. Preheat the oven to 425°F.

2. To a food processor or blender, add the shallot, thyme, rosemary, and garlic. Pulse to chop. Add the sage and parsley. Pulse lightly until mixed.

3. On a flat surface, place the chicken breast-side up. Carefully slide your fingers under the skin of each breast to separate the skin from the meat, creating a pocket. Do not remove the skin from the chicken.

4. Turn the chicken onto its side. Repeat the process of lifting up the skin on the thighs.

5. Stuff an equal amount of the herb mixture under the skin of the breasts and thighs. Place the chicken into a baking dish.

6. Pour the olive oil over the herbed chicken. Massage it into the skin. If any herb mixture is left, spread it over the outside of the chicken.

7. Place the baking dish in the preheated oven. Bake for 15 minutes. Remove the pan from the oven.

8. Arrange the jicama around the chicken, and season with salt and pepper. Return the pan to the oven. Reduce the heat to 375°F. Cook the chicken for 1 hour, or until the internal temperature reaches 165°F.

9. Remove the chicken from the oven. Allow the chicken to rest for at least 15 minutes before carving.

PERFECT
POULTRY

SPINACH AND BACON STUFFED CHICKEN THIGHS

SERVES 4
PREP TIME: 15 MINUTES ▪ COOK TIME: 35 MINUTES ▪ TOTAL TIME: 50 MINUTES

Chicken thighs are a great cut of meat to enjoy on the keto diet, especially when stuffed with delicious ingredients. This recipe highlights the combination of bacon and spinach for a rich, hearty meal. Served with a light salad and a citrusy vinaigrette, this is a great meal to make for dinner and save for lunch the next day.

5 bacon slices

2 tablespoons butter

1½ cups spinach

1 teaspoon minced garlic

¾ cup cream cheese, at room temperature

1 pound boneless chicken thighs

¼ cup shredded Swiss cheese, divided

¼ teaspoon salt

¼ teaspoon freshly ground black pepper

PERFECT
POULTRY

PER SERVING
RATIO: 4:1
CALORIES: 527
TOTAL FAT: 44.1g
CARBS: 2.4g
NET CARBS: 2.4g
FIBER: 0g
PROTEIN: 29.3g

1. Preheat the oven to 425°F.

2. On a baking sheet, place the bacon slices about ½ inch apart. Put the sheet in the preheated oven. Cook for 10 to 15 minutes, or until crispy. Set aside to cool. Maintain the oven temperature.

3. In large skillet over medium-high heat, melt the butter. Add the spinach and garlic. Cook until the spinach wilts, about 2 minutes. Remove the spinach from the skillet. Set aside.

4. Chop the cooled bacon into small pieces.

5. In a large bowl, mix together the cream cheese, sautéed spinach, and chopped bacon.

6. On a flat surface, lay out the chicken thighs. Spread the meat open so the thighs lay flat. Place an equal portion of the cream cheese mixture on each piece of chicken.

7. Top each with the Swiss cheese, equally divided.

8. Close the thighs. Secure with toothpicks. Season with the salt and pepper. Place the chicken thighs in a baking dish.

9. Put the baking dish into the preheated oven. Bake for about 18 minutes. With a meat thermometer, check the internal temperature. It should reach 165°F before serving.

TIME SAVING TIP: Use microwavable spinach and precooked bacon to make this dish in a flash. Look for pre-chopped spinach and thick-cut bacon. Most precooked bacon is very thin and not substantial in flavor, so make sure to buy a quality brand for the best results.

PERFECT POULTRY

FETA AND OLIVE STUFFED CHICKEN THIGHS

SERVES 4

PREP TIME: 15 MINUTES — COOK TIME: 20 MINUTES — TOTAL TIME: 35 MINUTES

For a Mediterranean vibe, try this feta and olive stuffed chicken recipe. Great on their own or served with Zucchini Noodles (page 121), these chicken thighs are bursting with Greek flavor. Top with extra feta for a cheesier bite.

1 cup crumbled feta cheese

¼ cup shredded Swiss cheese

1 teaspoon minced garlic

1 tablespoon olive oil

¼ cup olives, chopped

1 pound boneless chicken thighs

¼ teaspoon salt

¼ teaspoon freshly ground black pepper

PER SERVING
RATIO: 4:1
CALORIES: 407
TOTAL FAT: 31.3g
CARBS: 2.7g
NET CARBS: 2.3g
FIBER: 0.4g
PROTEIN: 27.3g

1. Preheat the oven to 425°F.

2. In a large bowl, mix together the feta cheese, Swiss cheese, garlic, olive oil, and olives.

3. On a flat surface, lay out the chicken thighs. Spread the meat open so the thighs lay flat. Place an equal portion of the feta mixture on each piece of chicken. Close the thighs. Secure with toothpicks. Season with the salt and pepper.

4. Place the chicken in a baking dish. Put the dish into the preheated oven and bake for about 18 minutes. With a meat thermometer, check the internal temperature. It should reach 165°F before serving.

CHICKEN THIGHS WITH LEMON CREAM SAUCE

SERVES 4

PREP TIME: 15 MINUTES ▪ COOK TIME: 20 MINUTES ▪ TOTAL TIME: 35 MINUTES

A creamy sauce is tempered with lemon in this simple recipe. It's best served with flavorful vegetables, like asparagus. Adjust the amount of lemon to suit your palate. If you enjoy this sauce, double the ingredients to have extra on hand for topping omelets or eggs at breakfast.

1 tablespoon butter

1 tablespoon minced shallots

1 cup sour cream

2 tablespoons freshly squeezed lemon juice

½ teaspoon salt, divided

¼ teaspoon freshly ground black pepper, divided

1 pound bone-in chicken thighs

1. Preheat the oven to 425°F.

2. In a large skillet over medium-low heat, melt the butter. Add the shallots. Cook for 3 to 4 minutes, or until tender. Decrease the heat to low. Add the sour cream, lemon juice, ¼ teaspoon of salt, and ⅛ teaspoon of pepper. Mix well to combine. Refrigerate until ready to serve.

3. Season the chicken with the remaining ¼ teaspoon of salt and ⅛ teaspoon of pepper.

4. Place the chicken into a baking dish and into the preheated oven. Bake for about 18 minutes. With a meat thermometer, check the internal temperature. It should reach 165°F.

5. Plate the chicken, spooning an equal amount of lemon cream sauce on each thigh.

PERFECT POULTRY

PER SERVING

RATIO: 4:1

CALORIES: 393

TOTAL FAT: 32g

CARBS: 3.1g

NET CARBS: 3.1g

FIBER: 0g

PROTEIN: 22.1g

CHICKEN PICCATA

SERVES 4

PREP TIME: 10 MINUTES • COOK TIME: 15 MINUTES • TOTAL TIME: 25 MINUTES

An Italian restaurant classic gets the keto treatment in this dish. The unique flavor of the capers and lemon juice pairs well with the chicken and white wine. Traditionally made with chicken breast, this recipe calls for chicken thighs to increase the amount of fat.

1 pound boneless chicken thighs

¼ teaspoon salt

⅛ teaspoon freshly ground black pepper

¼ cup olive oil

½ cup dry white wine

1 tablespoon freshly squeezed lemon juice

1 garlic clove, minced

1 tablespoon capers, chopped

3 tablespoons chopped fresh parsley

PERFECT POULTRY

PER SERVING
RATIO: 4:1
CALORIES: 377
TOTAL FAT: 29.7g
CARBS: 1.4g
NET CARBS: 1.4g
FIBER: 0g
PROTEIN: 20.3g

1. On a flat surface, flatten the chicken thighs with a meat tenderizer until they are ¼ inch thick. Season with the salt and pepper.

2. In a large skillet over medium heat, heat the olive oil for about 1 minute. Place two chicken thighs in the pan. Cook for about 4 minutes per side. Remove to a plate. Repeat, two at a time, with the remaining thighs. Set aside.

3. Using the same skillet, increase the heat to high. Add the white wine, lemon juice, garlic, and capers. Stir the sauce, scraping any browned bits from the bottom of the pan. Bring to a boil. Cook for 1 minute.

4. Add the chicken back into the pan. Heat in the sauce for 1 minute.

5. Add the parsley and stir to incorporate before serving.

PERFECT PAIR TIP: Zucchini Noodles (page 121) are an easy pick to accompany this dish, which is usually served with pasta. Toss the noodles in a skillet with some olive oil and cook until al dente. Serve with the piccata sauce or a spoonful of sugar-free Pasta Sauce (page 224).

BAKED CHICKEN TENDERS

SERVES 4

PREP TIME: 15 MINUTES ▪ COOK TIME: 20 MINUTES ▪ TOTAL TIME: 35 MINUTES

Every kid's favorite meal gets a keto twist with a non-bread "breading" made from some surprising ingredients. Instead of bread crumbs, crushed pork rinds and Parmesan cheese create a crust that is both crunchy and crisp. Dip in Ranch Dressing (page 218) or Sugar-Free Ketchup (page 216) for a real childhood treat.

2 eggs

½ cup pork rinds, ground

½ cup shredded Parmesan cheese

1 teaspoon garlic powder

1 teaspoon onion powder

¼ teaspoon salt

⅛ teaspoon freshly ground black pepper

1 pound boneless chicken thighs, halved

1. Preheat the oven to 400°F.

2. Line a baking sheet with parchment paper.

3. In a medium bowl, beat the eggs.

4. In another medium bowl, combine the pork rinds, Parmesan cheese, garlic powder, onion powder, salt, and pepper.

5. Create a "breading" station: Line up the egg wash, then the pork rind mixture, then the baking sheet.

6. Take one thigh half and dredge thoroughly in the egg wash, then coat in the pork rind mixture, pressing the "breading" into the meat so it adheres. Place the "breaded" thigh on the baking sheet. Repeat with the remaining thigh halves.

7. Place the baking sheet in the preheated oven. Cook for 18 to 20 minutes, or until golden brown.

PERFECT POULTRY

PER SERVING

RATIO: 3:1

CALORIES: 489

TOTAL FAT: 32.9g

CARBS: 2.2g

NET CARBS: 2.2g

FIBER: 0g

PROTEIN: 45.8g

BUFFALO CHICKEN WINGS

SERVES 4

PREP TIME: 15 MINUTES ▪ COOK TIME: 50 MINUTES ▪ TOTAL TIME: 1 HOUR

These classic wings are perfect for football Sundays or weekend gatherings. Baked instead of fried, these wings also save time and the expense of oil. For a smoky flavor, cook the chicken for the same amount of time on the grill over medium heat.

1 tablespoon olive oil

1 teaspoon salt, divided

½ teaspoon freshly ground black pepper, divided

2 pounds chicken wings

¼ cup hot sauce

1 tablespoon butter, melted

¼ teaspoon cayenne pepper

1 cup Bleu Cheese Sauce (page 217) or Ranch Dressing (page 218), or purchased bottled dressing

PER SERVING

RATIO: 3:1

CALORIES: 507

TOTAL FAT: 23.4g

CARBS: 3.7g

NET CARBS: 3.7g

FIBER: 0g

PROTEIN: 66.5g

1. Preheat the oven to 400°F.

2. In a large bowl, mix together the olive oil, ½ teaspoon of salt, and ¼ teaspoon of black pepper. Add the wings and stir to coat.

3. Evenly divide the wings between two baking sheets. Place the sheets in the oven. Bake for 45 to 50 minutes, or until the outer skin is crispy.

4. In another large bowl, mix together the hot sauce, butter, cayenne pepper, the remaining ½ teaspoon of salt, and remaining ¼ teaspoon of black pepper. Add the cooked wings. Toss them in the sauce for 1 minute to coat.

5. Serve with Bleu Cheese Sauce (page 217) or Ranch Dressing (page 218).

GREEN-CHILE CHICKEN ENCHILADA CASSEROLE

SERVES 8

PREP TIME: 30 MINUTES ▪ COOK TIME: 45 MINUTES ▪ TOTAL TIME: 1½ HOURS

Mild but flavorful green chiles blend with a creamy enchilada sauce in this tasty casserole that gets made at least once a month at my house. Sprinkled with strips of low-carb tortillas, this dish also captures the flavor of traditional enchiladas but without the high amount of carbs.

3 cups chicken broth

1½ pounds boneless chicken thighs

2 cups chopped fresh roasted green chiles, or canned

1 cup sour cream

2 cups shredded Monterey Jack cheese

½ cup diced onion

1 tablespoon minced garlic

½ teaspoon salt

½ teaspoon freshly ground black pepper

¼ teaspoon cayenne pepper

1 tablespoon olive oil

1 bunch fresh cilantro, chopped

2 low-carb tortillas cut into ½-inch-wide strips

PER SERVING

RATIO: 3:1

CALORIES: 413

TOTAL FAT: 26.9g

CARBS: 8.3g

NET CARBS: 6.2g

FIBER: 2.1g

PROTEIN: 33.1g

1. Preheat the oven to 400°F.

2. To a large pot over high heat, add the chicken broth. Bring to a boil. Reduce the heat to a simmer. Add the chicken thighs. Cook for 12 minutes. Remove the thighs and set aside to cool. Once cooled, shred the chicken into bite-size pieces. Transfer to a large bowl.

3. To the shredded chicken, add the green chiles, sour cream, Monterey Jack cheese, onion, garlic, salt, black pepper, and cayenne pepper. Mix thoroughly to combine.

4. In a medium skillet over medium-high heat, heat the olive oil for 1 minute. Add the tortilla strips and crisp for 2 to 3 minutes. Stir to avoid burning.

5. Transfer the chicken mixture to a large baking dish. Apply the cilantro liberally to the top of the chicken mixture, then add the tortilla strips.

6. Place the dish in the preheated oven. Cook for 15 to 20 minutes, or until golden brown.

7. Remove from the oven. Cool the casserole for 5 minutes before serving.

BACON-WRAPPED JALAPEÑO CHICKEN

SERVES 4

PREP TIME: 30 MINUTES ⚊ COOK TIME: 20 MINUTES ⚊ TOTAL TIME: 55 MINUTES

These chicken breasts get a healthy dose of spice from the chopped jalapeño, while the cream cheese mellows the heat. Serve with a side of Cauliflower Mac and Cheese (page 96).

4 (4-ounce) boneless chicken breasts

¾ cup cream cheese, at room temperature

4 jalapeño peppers, halved

1 teaspoon onion powder

2 garlic cloves, minced

8 bacon slices

¼ teaspoon salt

⅛ teaspoon freshly ground black pepper

2 tablespoons olive oil

PER SERVING

RATIO: 3:1

CALORIES: 586

TOTAL FAT: 42.2g

CARBS: 3.8g

NET CARBS: 3.3g

FIBER: 0.5g

PROTEIN: 46.9g

1. Preheat the oven to 400°F.

2. On a flat surface, cut each chicken breast in half horizontally. Do not cut all the way through the other side. Open the breasts flat.

3. Spread an equal amount of cream cheese over each of the butterflied breasts.

4. Top each with two jalapeño halves. Sprinkle with onion powder and garlic. Fold the breasts closed. Wrap each breast with two bacon slices. Secure with toothpicks. Season the outside of the breasts with the salt and pepper.

5. Place the bacon-wrapped chicken in a baking pan. Drizzle with the olive oil.

6. Put the pan into the preheated oven. Bake the chicken for 20 minutes, or until the internal temperature is 165°F.

7. Remove the pan from the oven. Allow the chicken to rest for 2 to 3 minutes. Remove the toothpicks from the meat and serve.

COOKING TIP: Double this recipe and freeze each bacon-wrapped chicken breast individually for a quick meal on a busy night. Heat the oven to 400°F and cook the frozen breast for an extra 5 to 7 minutes (25 to 27 minutes total). If you defrost the chicken first, keep to the original cooking time.

CILANTRO CHILI CHICKEN SKEWERS

SERVES 4

PREP TIME: 15 MINUTES · COOK TIME: 10 MINUTES · TOTAL TIME: 40 MINUTES

Cilantro and spicy chili come together on these tangy chicken skewers mixed with peppers and onions. Full of flavor from the fresh cilantro, this dish can be made by using the broil setting in your oven or over medium-high heat on the grill. Enjoy with a low-carb tortilla or a scoop of Cauliflower "Rice" (page 98).

1 cup fresh cilantro, chopped

2 tablespoons olive oil

¼ cup red chili paste

2 tablespoons soy sauce

2 garlic cloves, minced

1 teaspoon onion powder

1 teaspoon minced fresh ginger

¼ teaspoon freshly ground black pepper

1 pound boneless chicken thighs cut into 1-inch cubes

1 onion, roughly chopped

2 red bell peppers, roughly chopped

PER SERVING

RATIO: 3:1

CALORIES: 355

TOTAL FAT: 25g

CARBS: 11.2g

NET CARBS: 9g

FIBER: 2.2g

PROTEIN: 21.7g

1. Preheat the oven to broil.

2. In a large bowl, combine the cilantro, olive oil, red chili paste, soy sauce, garlic, onion powder, ginger, and black pepper.

3. Add the thigh meat. Toss to coat. Refrigerate for 15 minutes to marinate.

4. Remove the chicken from the refrigerator. Skewer the chicken cubes, alternating with the onions and peppers between each piece.

5. Place a foil-lined baking sheet on the lowest oven rack.

6. Lay the chicken skewers directly on the middle rack above the baking sheet, perpendicular to the rack. Cook for 3 minutes. Turn the skewers over and cook for 3 minutes more. Turn the skewers again, and cook for 4 minutes more. With a meat thermometer, check the internal temperature. When it reaches 165°F, remove from the oven to cool.

7. Serve on the skewers or remove the meat and vegetables from the skewers prior to plating.

AVOCADO CHICKEN BURGER

SERVES 4

PREP TIME: 5 MINUTES ▪ COOK TIME: 15 MINUTES ▪ TOTAL TIME: 20 MINUTES

Possibly one of the simplest dinner recipes for the keto diet is an avocado chicken burger. Packed with healthy fats, avocado is the ultimate addition to any protein-based meal. Top these burgers with alfalfa sprouts and goat cheese or a slice of Swiss—however you serve them, they're a palate pleaser.

1 pound ground chicken

½ cup almond flour

2 garlic cloves, minced

1 teaspoon onion powder

¼ teaspoon salt

⅛ teaspoon freshly ground black pepper

1 avocado, diced

2 tablespoons olive oil

4 low-carb buns or lettuce wraps (optional)

PER SERVING
(1 PATTY)
RATIO: 3:1
CALORIES: 413
TOTAL FAT: 25.7g
CARBS: 7.9g
NET CARBS: 2.9g
FIBER: 5g
PROTEIN: 33.9g

1. In a large bowl, mix together the ground chicken, almond flour, garlic, onion powder, salt, and pepper.

2. Add the avocado, gently incorporating into the meat while forming four patties. Set aside.

3. In a large skillet over medium heat, heat the olive oil for about 1 minute. Add the patties to the skillet. Cook for about 8 minutes per side, or until golden brown and cooked through.

4. Serve on a low-carb bun, in a lettuce wrap (if using), or on its own.

INGREDIENT TIP: If using alfalfa sprouts, it's important to note that they can sometimes carry harmful bacteria. To avoid this problem, wash them a minimum of two times before consuming.

CURRIED CHICKEN

SERVES 4

PREP TIME: 10 MINUTES ▪ COOK TIME: 25 MINUTES ▪ TOTAL TIME: 35 MINUTES

Rich coconut milk is spiced with curry powder in this excellent chicken curry recipe. Accompanied by bamboo shoots and onion, the chicken thighs absorb the deep flavors of paprika and ginger for a bright, crisp curry. Serve over crisped Cauliflower "Rice" (page 98) or, for something different, Zucchini Noodles (page 121).

4 tablespoons coconut oil

¼ cup diced onion

1 cup bamboo shoots

1 pound boneless chicken thighs, diced

1 teaspoon minced fresh ginger

1 tablespoon curry powder

1 tablespoon paprika

1¼ cups coconut milk

¼ cup heavy (whipping) cream

¼ teaspoon salt

⅛ teaspoon freshly ground black pepper

1. In a large skillet over medium-high heat, heat the coconut oil for about 1 minute. Add the onion, bamboo shoots, and chicken meat. Cook for 5 minutes.

2. Stir in the ginger, curry powder, and paprika. Continue cooking for 2 to 3 minutes more.

3. Add the coconut milk and heavy cream. Reduce the heat to medium-low. Simmer for about 15 minutes. Season with salt and pepper.

4. Serve over Cauliflower "Rice" (page 98) or Zucchini Noodles (page 121).

PERFECT POULTRY

PER SERVING

RATIO: 4:1

CALORIES: 582

TOTAL FAT: 51.9g

CARBS: 9.2g

NET CARBS: 5.3g

FIBER: 3.9g

PROTEIN: 23.5g

JAMAICAN JERK CHICKEN

SERVES 4

PREP TIME: 10 MINUTES ▪ COOK TIME: 1 HOUR ▪

TOTAL TIME: 5 HOURS, INCLUDES MARINATING TIME

A taste of the islands is not far away with this authentic jerk chicken recipe. Traditionally made with sugar, this jerk marinade is keto friendly and can be made in advance or doubled for multiple uses. While most jerk chicken is made over an open flame, the addition of some liquid smoke does that work for you while the chicken roasts in the oven.

PER SERVING
RATIO: 3:1
CALORIES: 557
TOTAL FAT: 36g
CARBS: 4g
NET CARBS: 3.1g
FIBER: 0.9g
PROTEIN: 42.8g

1 onion, finely chopped

½ cup finely chopped scallions

3 tablespoons soy sauce

1 tablespoon apple cider vinegar

1 tablespoon olive oil

2 teaspoons chopped fresh thyme

2 teaspoons Splenda, or other sugar substitute

1 teaspoon liquid smoke

1 teaspoon salt

1 teaspoon allspice

1 teaspoon cayenne pepper

1 teaspoon freshly ground black pepper

½ teaspoon nutmeg

½ teaspoon cinnamon

1 whole chicken, quartered

1. In a medium bowl, mix together the onion, scallion, soy sauce, cider vinegar, olive oil, thyme, Splenda, liquid smoke, salt, allspice, cayenne pepper, black pepper, nutmeg, and cinnamon.

2. In a large dish, place the chicken pieces skin-side down. Pour the marinade over it. Marinate covered, in the refrigerator, for at least 4 hours.

3. When ready to cook, preheat the oven to 425°F.

4. Place the baking dish with the chicken into the preheated oven. Cook for 30 minutes.

5. Remove the baking dish from the oven. Turn the chicken skin-side up. Return the pan to the oven. Cook for 20 to 30 minutes more, or until the internal temperature checked with a meat thermometer reaches 165°F.

6. Cool the chicken for 5 minutes before cutting and serving.

SESAME BROILED CHICKEN THIGHS

SERVES 4

PREP TIME: 5 MINUTES ▪ COOK TIME: 20 MINUTES ▪ TOTAL TIME: 25 MINUTES

If you crave Chinese takeout as much as I do, whip up these quick and delicious sesame chicken thighs instead of reaching for your phone. The deep, nutty flavor of sesame oil tempers the sweetness of the maple syrup in this sweet and savory dish. I like to serve these with a steamed and buttered vegetable like broccoli and Cauliflower "Rice" (page 98) for a filling meal. Add optional sesame seeds for a presentation to rival your local takeout joint.

4 bone-in, skin-on chicken thighs

¼ teaspoon salt

¼ teaspoon freshly ground black pepper

2 tablespoons soy sauce

2 tablespoons sugar-free maple syrup

1 tablespoon sesame oil

1 teaspoon minced garlic

1 teaspoon red wine vinegar

½ teaspoon crushed red pepper flakes

PER SERVING
(1 THIGH)

RATIO: 3:1

CALORIES: 360

TOTAL FAT: 26g

CARBS: 2.2g

NET CARBS: 2.2g

FIBER: 0g

PROTEIN: 27.1g

1. Season the chicken with the salt and pepper. Set aside.

2. In a bowl large enough to hold the chicken, combine the soy sauce, maple syrup, sesame oil, garlic, vinegar, and red pepper flakes. Reserve about one-quarter of the sauce.

3. Add the chicken thighs to the bowl, skin-side up. Submerge in the soy sauce. Refrigerate to marinate for at least 15 minutes.

4. Preheat the oven to broil.

5. Remove the chicken from the refrigerator. Place the thighs skin-side down in the baking dish.

6. Place the dish in the preheated oven, about six inches from the broiler. Broil for 5 to 6 minutes with the oven door slightly ajar. Turn the chicken skin-side up. Broil for about 2 minutes more.

7. Turn the chicken again so it is now skin-side down. Move the baking dish to the bottom rack of the oven. Close the oven door and broil for another 6 to 8 minutes.

(continued)

8. Turn the chicken again to skin-side up. Baste with the reserved sauce. Close the oven door and broil for 2 minutes more.

9. Remove the chicken from the oven. With a meat thermometer, check the internal temperature. It should reach at least 165°F.

10. Cool the chicken for 5 minutes before serving.

PERFECT POULTRY

FRUGAL FRIENDLY TIP: On keto, bone-in chicken thighs are preferable to boneless chicken thighs. Bone-in chicken thighs are often cheaper and sold in bulk. Stock up on bone-in thighs and, if a recipe arises where you need boneless chicken, debone the thighs and reserve the bones for homemade chicken stock.

BACON RANCH CHEESY CHICKEN BREASTS

SERVES 4

PREP TIME: 10 MINUTES · COOK TIME: 55 MINUTES · TOTAL TIME: 1 HOUR

You know what they say: Everything is better with bacon. That saying is even more true when bacon is served with Ranch Dressing (page 218). Topped with ranch, bacon, and cheese, these chicken breasts are moist and tender, and perfect for an easy weeknight meal. Serve with a lighter side dish, like steamed vegetables.

Cooking spray for the baking dish

3 tablespoons olive oil

4 boneless chicken breasts

½ teaspoon salt

¼ teaspoon freshly ground black pepper

1 tablespoon garlic powder

8 bacon slices

4 tablespoons butter

4 tablespoons Ranch Dressing (page 218), or purchased bottled dressing

½ cup shredded Cheddar cheese, divided

½ cup shredded mozzarella cheese

½ cup grated Parmesan cheese

½ teaspoon dried parsley

PER SERVING
(1 CHICKEN BREAST)

RATIO: 4:1

CALORIES: 674

TOTAL FAT: 52.3g

CARBS: 4.2g

NET CARBS: 3.9g

FIBER: 0.3g

PROTEIN: 46.5g

1. Preheat the oven to 350°F and prepare a baking dish with cooking spray.

2. In a large skillet over medium-high heat, heat the olive oil for about 1 minute. Season the chicken breasts with the salt, pepper, and garlic powder. Add them to the skillet. Sear each breast for 5 minutes per side.

3. Slice the bacon into small pieces, about 12 cuts per slice.

4. Place the chicken into the prepared dish. Spread 1 tablespoon of butter and 1 tablespoon of ranch dressing over each breast.

5. Top the chicken with the bacon, covering each breast completely.

6. Place the dish in the preheated oven. Bake for 30 minutes. Remove from the oven.

7. Sprinkle equal amounts of the Cheddar, mozzarella, and Parmesan cheeses over the bacon-topped breasts. Season with the dried parsley. Return the dish to the oven.

8. Bake for another 10 to 12 minutes, or until the cheese melts.

9. Remove the dish from the oven. Allow to rest for about 2 minutes before serving.

CHICKEN FAJITA STUFFED BELL PEPPERS

SERVES 6

PREP TIME: 10 MINUTES ▪ COOK TIME: 50 MINUTES ▪ TOTAL TIME: 1 HOUR

Eat in tonight with these delicious Mexican-inspired stuffed bell peppers. Rich with flavor from homemade fajita seasoning, you can adapt these with other vegetables or different meats depending on your mood. Try a dollop of sour cream and a dash of chili powder on top for added presentation value.

½ cup butter, divided

1 pound boneless chicken thighs

½ cup chopped onion

1½ cups Cauliflower "Rice" (page 98)

¼ cup chopped scallions

½ cup chicken broth

2 teaspoons chili powder

1 teaspoon paprika

1 teaspoon salt

½ teaspoon cumin

½ teaspoon garlic powder

¼ teaspoon dried oregano

¼ teaspoon cayenne pepper (optional)

6 bell peppers, tops removed and seeded

1 cup shredded Mexican cheese blend

PER SERVING
(1 PEPPER)
RATIO: 3:1
CALORIES: 419
TOTAL FAT: 28.3g
CARBS: 11.8g
NET CARBS: 7.8g
FIBER: 4g
PROTEIN: 29.2g

1. Preheat the oven to 350°F.

2. In a large skillet over medium-high heat, heat 6 tablespoons of butter. Add the chicken. Sear for 3 to 4 minutes on each side. Cover. Reduce the heat to medium-low. Cook for another 10 to 12 minutes. Check the chicken for doneness. Set aside to cool.

3. Once cooled, shred the chicken into small pieces. Set aside.

4. In a large skillet over medium-high heat, melt the remaining 2 tablespoons of butter. Add the onion. Cook for 3 to 4 minutes, until translucent.

5. Add the Cauliflower "Rice" (page 98), shredded chicken, scallions, chicken broth, chili powder, paprika, salt, cumin, garlic powder, dried oregano, and cayenne pepper (if using).

6. Slice a thin piece from the bottom of each bell pepper so it will not tip over. Place the peppers open-side up on a baking sheet.

7. Fill each bell pepper with an equal amount of the chicken mixture.

8. Top evenly with the Mexican cheese blend.

9. Place the sheet in the oven. Bake for about 30 minutes, or until the cheese browns.

TIP: The fillings and toppings for this fajita-inspired dish also make for excellent tacos. Try using the Cheesy Taco Shells (page 106) for a hand-held twist, and omit the chicken broth in the filling.

WHITE CHILI

SERVES 12

PREP TIME: 15 MINUTES ▪ COOK TIME: 6 HOURS ▪ TOTAL TIME: 7 HOURS

Nothing warms you up on a cold night like a warm bowl of chili. If beef chili just isn't your thing, this white chicken chili is sure to hit the spot. Green chiles are tempered with Cheddar cheese and sour cream but overall, this is a very mild chili. Add a jalapeño or serrano pepper to heighten the heat.

½ cup butter

2 cups chopped onion

2 cups peeled, cubed turnips

1½ cups diced red bell pepper

½ cup diced orange or yellow bell pepper

1 (3-ounce) can diced green chiles

4 garlic cloves, minced

2 pounds ground chicken

5 cups chicken broth

2 teaspoons chili powder (or to taste)

2 teaspoons cumin

2 teaspoons oregano

1 teaspoon cayenne pepper

1 teaspoon salt

1 teaspoon freshly ground black pepper

16 ounces sour cream

2 cups shredded Cheddar cheese

PER SERVING

RATIO: 3:1

CALORIES: 413

TOTAL FAT: 28.3g

CARBS: 8.4g

NET CARBS: 6.8g

FIBER: 1.6g

PROTEIN: 30.6g

1. In a large stockpot over medium-high heat, melt the butter. Add the onion. Sweat for 8 to 10 minutes, stirring occasionally.

2. Add the turnips, red bell pepper, orange bell pepper, green chiles, and garlic. Sauté for 5 to 6 minutes.

3. Add the ground chicken. Stir to break up the meat, browning on all sides for 6 to 8 minutes.

4. Pour in the chicken broth. Stir to combine.

5. Add the chili powder, cumin, oregano, and cayenne pepper. Bring to a boil. Reduce the heat to low.

6. Cook the chili for 6 to 8 hours, until reduced and thickened. Season with the salt and black pepper.

7. Serve with the sour cream and Cheddar cheese.

CHICKEN CORDON BLEU

SERVES 8

PREP TIME: 25 MINUTES ▪ COOK TIME: 30 MINUTES ▪ TOTAL TIME: 55 MINUTES

A restaurant classic gets the keto makeover with a surprise ingredient for the outer, crispy breading. Pork rinds substitute for bread crumbs to create a crunch that's not only unique but also extra flavorful. Serve with steamed vegetables or Cauliflower Mash (page 99) for a filling meal.

Cooking spray for the baking dish

18 ounces thinly sliced chicken thighs (about 8 pieces)

8 ounces pork rinds

¼ cup grated Parmesan cheese

½ teaspoon dried parsley

½ teaspoon dried oregano

½ teaspoon dried basil

¼ teaspoon dried rosemary

¼ teaspoon garlic powder

¼ teaspoon onion powder

¼ teaspoon crushed red pepper flakes

¼ teaspoon salt

¼ teaspoon freshly ground black pepper

2 eggs

3 ounces (3 slices) deli ham, halved, divided

2 ounces (3 slices) Swiss cheese, halved, divided

8 tablespoons (1 stick) butter, divided

PER SERVING
(1 CHICKEN ROLL)
RATIO: 3:1
CALORIES: 481
TOTAL FAT: 32.6g
CARBS: 1.6g
NET CARBS: 1.3g
FIBER: 0.3g
PROTEIN: 45.3g

1. Preheat the oven to 450°F.

2. Coat the baking dish with cooking spray.

3. On a flat surface, place the chicken thighs between two pieces of plastic wrap. Pound the chicken until the pieces are all about ¼ inch thick. Set aside.

4. In a food processor, pulse the pork rinds into a fine powder. Transfer to a large bowl.

5. To the ground pork rinds, add the Parmesan cheese, parsley, oregano, basil, rosemary, garlic powder, onion powder, red pepper flakes, salt, and pepper. Mix the coating thoroughly.

6. In a medium bowl, beat the eggs.

7. Set up a "breading" station: Line up the egg wash, then the pork rind mixture, then the prepared baking dish.

(continued)

8. On a flat surface, lay out each chicken breast. Top each breast with one-half slice of ham and one-half slice of Swiss cheese. Top each with 1 tablespoon of butter. Roll up each breast, finishing seam-side down.

9. Carefully dip one chicken roll into the egg wash, then coat completely with the pork rind mixture, pressing firmly so the "breading" adheres. Place the breaded chicken roll seam-side down into the prepared pan. Repeat the "breading" process with the remaining chicken rolls.

10. Place the pan in the oven. Bake for 25 to 30 minutes, until golden brown.

PERFECT POULTRY

CHICKEN PARMESAN

SERVES 6

PREP TIME: 20 MINUTES ▪ COOK TIME: 35 MINUTES ▪ TOTAL TIME: 55 MINUTES

Almond flour and Parmesan cheese combine to create the perfect coating for this keto Chicken Parmesan recipe. Topped with sugar-free Pasta Sauce (page 224) and melted mozzarella, this entrée pairs well with sautéed vegetables or Zucchini Noodles (page 121). Try this recipe with chicken thighs for added fat content.

3 large boneless chicken breasts, halved

¾ cup grated Parmesan cheese, divided

½ cup almond flour

1 teaspoon Italian seasoning

½ teaspoon garlic powder

¼ teaspoon salt

⅛ teaspoon freshly ground black pepper

1 egg

¼ cup olive oil

6 tablespoons sugar-free Pasta Sauce (page 224), divided

1 cup shredded mozzarella cheese, divided

1. Preheat the oven to 350°F.

2. Place the chicken between two pieces of plastic wrap. Pound the chicken and flatten until all pieces are about ½ inch thick.

3. In a medium bowl, mix ½ cup of Parmesan cheese, the almond flour, Italian seasoning, garlic powder, salt, and pepper.

4. In another bowl, beat the egg.

5. Set up a "breading" station: Line up the egg wash, then the Parmesan coating. Dip each piece of chicken into the egg wash, then thoroughly coat in the "breading." Set aside.

6. In a large skillet over medium-high heat, heat the olive oil for about 2 minutes. Add the "breaded" chicken. Cook for 5 to 7 minutes, or until browned on each side.

7. Remove from the skillet and place on a parchment-lined baking sheet.

8. Top with 1 tablespoon of Pasta Sauce (page 224) and divide the 1 cup of mozzarella cheese among the chicken. Sprinkle each with the remaining Parmesan cheese.

9. Place the baking sheet in the oven. Bake for 20 minutes, until the cheese is thoroughly melted.

PER SERVING
(½ CHICKEN BREAST WITH SAUCE AND CHEESE)

RATIO: 3:1

CALORIES: 469

TOTAL FAT: 29.8g

CARBS: 3.9g

NET CARBS: 2.6g

FIBER: 1.3g

PROTEIN: 43.9g

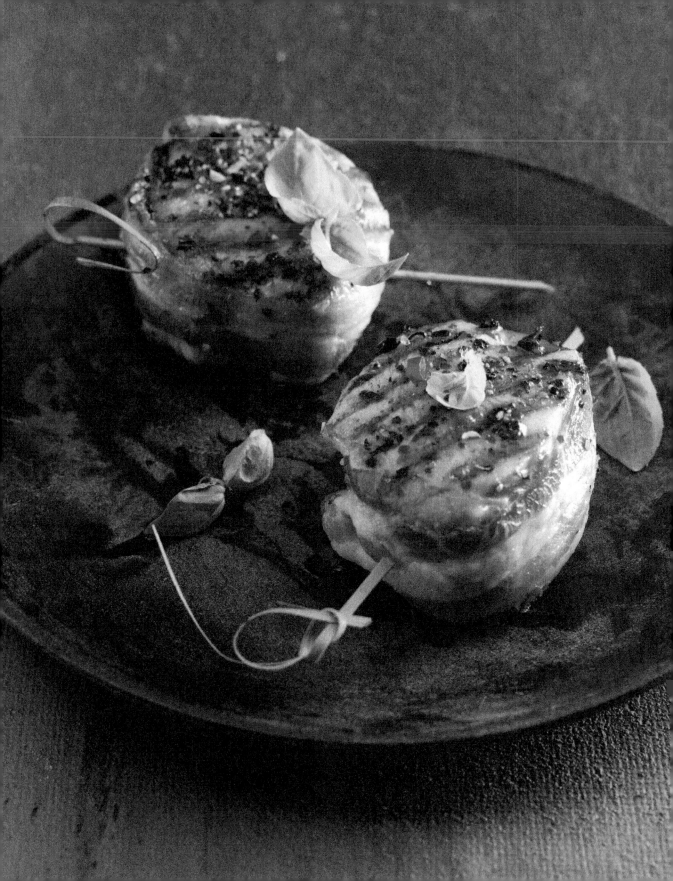

CHAPTER

MEATY MAINS

BACON-WRAPPED PORK LOIN

SERVES 4

PREP TIME: 10 MINUTES ▪ COOK TIME: 45 MINUTES ▪ TOTAL TIME: 1 HOUR

Wrapping pork tenderloin in more pork may seem redundant but you'll realize quickly after this dish starts baking what an impact the bacon wrap has on the overall flavor. In addition to the added flavor, the bacon helps keep the pork moist on the inside. Serve this with your favorite steamed vegetables and Cauliflower Mash (page 99).

PER SERVING
RATIO: 3:1
CALORIES: 518
TOTAL FAT: 29.9g
CARBS: 1.9g
NET CARBS: 1.9g
FIBER: 0g
PROTEIN: 57.3g

FOR THE RUB

1 teaspoon salt

1 teaspoon garlic powder

1 teaspoon onion powder

½ teaspoon smoked paprika

½ teaspoon dried basil

½ teaspoon dried thyme

½ teaspoon dried rosemary

½ teaspoon dried sage

½ teaspoon freshly ground black pepper

¼ teaspoon cayenne pepper

¼ teaspoon cumin

⅛ teaspoon cinnamon

⅛ teaspoon nutmeg

⅛ teaspoon cloves

FOR THE LOIN

2 pounds pork tenderloin

2 tablespoons olive oil

8 to 12 bacon slices

To make the rub

In a medium bowl, combine the salt, garlic powder, onion powder, paprika, basil, thyme, rosemary, sage, black pepper, cayenne pepper, cumin, cinnamon, nutmeg, and cloves. Stir to combine. Set aside.

To make the loin

1. Preheat the oven to 425°F.

2. Trim any excess fat or silverskin (a thin layer of connective tissue) from the pork. Coat the pork with the olive oil.

3. Liberally apply the rub to the pork, covering the entire loin. Set aside.

4. On a cutting board, lay out the bacon pieces side by side. Place the pork in the center of the bacon strips. Starting at one end, pull the edge of the bacon up and over the tenderloin diagonally. Repeat with the other side of the slice, crossing it over the first side. Repeat the process with the remaining bacon slices, tucking the free ends under the crisscrossed bacon slices as you go. Secure with toothpicks as needed.

5. Put the bacon-wrapped pork in a baking dish and place it in the preheated oven. Bake for 20 minutes. Lower the heat to 300°F and bake for another 20 minutes.

6. Use a meat thermometer inserted into the thickest part of the meat to check the temperature. Once it reaches 135°F, increase the heat to broil and crisp the bacon for 3 to 5 minutes.

7. Remove the pork from the oven. Cover with aluminum foil. Allow the meat to rest for at least 10 minutes so the juices set.

8. Slice and serve with your preferred sides.

INGREDIENT TIP: The amount of bacon you'll need depends on the length and overall size of the pork tenderloin. There should be enough bacon to go from tip to tip of the tenderloin.

COOKING TIP: While the USDA recommends cooking pork to a minimum of 145°F, meat continues to cook after it is removed from the heat. For a juicier, more tender pork loin, allow the meat to cook the additional 10°F while it is resting. If the meat does not reach 145°F after resting, return it to the heat.

STUFFED BONE-IN PORK CHOPS

SERVES 2

PREP TIME: 15 MINUTES • COOK TIME: 20 MINUTES • TOTAL TIME: 35 MINUTES

Much like a bone-in rib-eye steak, a bone-in pork chop is a great cut of meat to use when you want to ensure a moist, perfectly cooked meal. Stuffed with garlicky spinach and Muenster cheese, this recipe is sure to satisfy.

FOR THE STUFFING

2 tablespoons olive oil, divided

1 teaspoon minced garlic

3 tablespoons finely chopped onion

⅓ cup spinach

2 ounces Muenster cheese, shredded

1 egg, beaten

FOR THE PORK CHOPS

2 (6- to 8-ounce) bone-in pork chops

½ teaspoon salt

¼ teaspoon finely ground black pepper

PER SERVING
(1 STUFFED
PORK CHOP)
RATIO: 3:1
CALORIES: 591
TOTAL FAT: 44.5g
CARBS: 4g
NET CARBS: 2.6g
FIBER: 1.4g
PROTEIN: 45.5g

To make the stuffing

1. In a large oven-safe skillet over medium-high heat, heat 1 tablespoon of olive oil for 1 minute. Add the garlic and sauté until fragrant, about 1 minute. Add the onion and spinach. Lower the heat to medium and cook for 2 to 3 minutes. Transfer the mixture to a small bowl to cool.

2. Once cooled, add the Muenster cheese and the egg. Mix well to combine.

To make the pork chops

1. Preheat the oven to 375°F.

2. On a flat surface, cut the pork chops through the middle horizontally to the bone. Open the meat up like a butterfly. Stuff half of the spinach mixture into each pork chop. Fold the chop together over the stuffing and secure the edges with toothpicks, if necessary. Season with the salt and pepper.

3. In the large oven-safe skillet, heat the remaining tablespoon of olive oil over medium-high heat. Place the chops into the skillet and sear each side for 2 minutes. Once seared, remove the skillet from the heat and place it into the preheated oven. Bake for 15 minutes, or until the internal temperature reaches 150°F.

4. Serve with your preferred side dishes.

ROSEMARY BALSAMIC PORK MEDALLIONS

SERVES 3

PREP TIME: 15 MINUTES ▪ COOK TIME: 20 MINUTES ▪ TOTAL TIME: 35 MINUTES

Succulent and flavorful pork medallions are seasoned with fresh rosemary and balsamic vinegar in this recipe. The herbaceous rosemary cuts through the usually thick flavor of the balsamic vinegar for a perfect pairing. Serve with Cauliflower Mash (page 99) or steamed asparagus for a complete meal.

1 (1-pound) pork tenderloin, sliced into 1½-inch-thick medallions

¼ teaspoon salt

¼ teaspoon freshly ground black pepper

2 tablespoons olive oil

4 tablespoons butter, divided

1 garlic clove, minced

1 shallot, minced

3 tablespoons balsamic vinegar

1 teaspoon soy sauce

4 fresh rosemary sprigs

4 fresh thyme sprigs

MEATY MAINS

PER SERVING

RATIO: 3:1

CALORIES: 458

TOTAL FAT: 30.7g

CARBS: 4.8g

NET CARBS: 2.5g

FIBER: 2.3g

PROTEIN: 40.4g

1. Preheat the oven to 475°F.

2. Season each medallion with the salt and pepper.

3. In a large oven-safe skillet over medium-high heat, heat the olive oil and 1 tablespoon of butter for 1 minute. Add the garlic and shallot and sauté until fragrant, about 1 minute. Add the pork medallions to the skillet. Sear on each side for about 2 minutes.

4. Add the balsamic vinegar, soy sauce, rosemary, thyme, and the remaining 3 tablespoons of butter to the skillet. Stir to combine. Spoon the balsamic mixture over the pork. Bring to a simmer and cook for about 2 minutes.

5. Remove the skillet from the heat and place it into the preheated oven. Bake for 5 minutes. Flip the medallions and spoon the balsamic mixture over each piece. Continue baking for an additional 5 minutes, or until the internal temperature reaches 150°F.

6. Remove from the oven and allow the pork to rest for 2 to 3 minutes before serving.

7. Serve with your preferred sides and any remaining balsamic sauce from the pan.

PULLED PORK WITH CABBAGE SLAW

SERVES 8

PREP TIME: 30 MINUTES • COOK TIME: 8½ HOURS • TOTAL TIME: 9 HOURS

A true Southern classic, pulled pork is one of the easiest dishes to prepare in a slow cooker while you're at work. Served with a light cabbage slaw, this recipe can be eaten as is or with homemade Barbecue Sauce (page 214). Enjoy this delicious pork and slaw with a fork or pair with a low-carb bun for a treat. If you do not have a slow cooker, cook the pork in a Dutch oven in a 200°F oven for the same amount of time.

PER SERVING
RATIO: 3:1
CALORIES: 750
TOTAL FAT: 58.8g
CARBS: 7.3g
NET CARBS: 5.5g
FIBER: 1.8g
PROTEIN: 44.4g

FOR THE SLAW

¾ cup shredded cabbage

¼ cup shredded carrot

⅛ cup sliced scallions

3 tablespoons mayonnaise

1 teaspoon mustard

¼ teaspoon salt

¼ teaspoon freshly ground black pepper

FOR THE RUB

4 tablespoons stevia, or other sugar substitute

1 tablespoon paprika

2 teaspoons garlic powder

2 teaspoons onion powder

2 teaspoons mustard powder

1 teaspoon ground cumin

1 teaspoon salt

1 teaspoon freshly ground black pepper

½ teaspoon chili powder

FOR THE PORK

1 (4- to 5-pound) boneless pork shoulder roast

2½ tablespoons olive oil

¾ cup light beer

3 tablespoons apple cider vinegar

3 tablespoons tomato paste

8 low-carb buns or lettuce wraps (optional)

To make the slaw

In a large bowl, combine the cabbage, carrots, scallions, mayonnaise, mustard, salt, and pepper. Mix thoroughly. Refrigerate until ready to serve.

To make the rub

In a medium bowl, mix together the stevia, paprika, garlic powder, onion powder, mustard powder, cumin, salt, pepper, and chili powder.

To make the pork

1. Cover the pork shoulder with the rub, massaging it thoroughly into the meat.

2. In a large skillet over medium-high heat, heat the olive oil for 1 minute. Add the pork to the skillet, browning on all sides for about 3 minutes per side. Once browned, remove the pork from the skillet and set aside.

3. Pour the beer into the skillet and scrape the bottom of the pan to loosen any browned bits. Remove the skillet from the heat and pour the drippings into a large slow cooker.

4. To the slow cooker, add the apple cider vinegar and tomato paste. Whisk to combine with the pork drippings.

5. Place the pork in the slow cooker and spoon some of the liquid over it. Cover. Cook on low for 8 hours. Insert a meat thermometer into the center of the pork to check the internal temperature. It should be between 180°F and 200°F.

6. Remove the pork from the slow cooker and place it in a large bowl to cool.

7. In a large skillet over high heat, add the remaining liquid from the slow cooker and bring to a boil. Lower the heat to medium-low and reduce the liquid by at least half over the next 10 minutes.

8. Using two forks, shred the cooled pork until you have bite-size chunks.

9. Pour the reduced liquid over the meat. Mix until it is coated evenly.

10. Serve the shredded pork with the slaw on its own, or on a low-carb bun or a lettuce wrap (if using).

BARBECUE PORK RIBS

SERVES 5

PREP TIME: 4½ HOURS • COOK TIME: 1 HOUR • TOTAL TIME: 5½ HOURS

Nothing says backyard barbecue like a plate of ribs. Skip the hassle of hauling out the grill with this oven preparation. Covered in your favorite sugar-free barbecue sauce or served with just the rub, these ribs pair well with Cauliflower Mac and Cheese (page 96) or cabbage slaw.

PER SERVING
RATIO: 4:1
CALORIES: 612
TOTAL FAT: 53.7g
CARBS: 2.3g
NET CARBS: 1.8g
FIBER: 0.5g
PROTEIN: 29.4g

FOR THE RUB

¼ cup olive oil

2 garlic cloves, minced

1 shallot, minced

1 teaspoon cumin

1 teaspoon paprika

1 teaspoon chili powder

1 teaspoon salt

½ teaspoon cayenne pepper

½ teaspoon freshly ground black pepper

¼ teaspoon ground ginger

FOR THE RIBS

2 pounds baby back pork rib racks

Barbecue Sauce (page 214), or purchased sugar-free barbecue sauce (optional)

To make the rub

In a blender or food processor, add the olive oil, garlic, shallot, cumin, paprika, chili powder, salt, cayenne pepper, black pepper, and ginger. Mix until thoroughly incorporated.

To make the ribs

1. On a flat surface, cut the rib racks into quarters and arrange on a baking sheet. Cover the ribs evenly with the rub, massaging it into the meat. Refrigerate the ribs to marinate for at least 4 hours.

2. Preheat the oven to 300°F.

3. Place the ribs in the oven. Cook for 1 hour, 10 minutes.

4. Remove the ribs from the oven. Allow them to cool for 2 to 3 minutes before slicing.

5. Sauce the ribs with your favorite sugar-free barbecue sauce (if using).

GRILLED HANGER STEAK WITH CILANTRO CREMA

SERVES 3
PREP TIME: 15 MINUTES ▪ COOK TIME: 20 MINUTES ▪ TOTAL TIME: 45 MINUTES

Hanger steak may not be a familiar cut; it's often referred to as the "butcher's steak" or "butcher's cut" since it's so flavorful that butchers often reserve it for themselves. Nowadays you can find hanger steak at most meat markets. If you can't locate it, just ask the butcher, who may have some in the back. Paired with an herbaceous cilantro crema, this steak cooked rare is one that you'll never forget.

FOR THE CILANTRO CREMA

¼ cup sliced scallions

¼ cup fresh cilantro, chopped

1 garlic clove

1 teaspoon grated lime rind

1½ teaspoons freshly squeezed lime juice

3 tablespoons mayonnaise

3 tablespoons sour cream

¼ teaspoon salt

FOR THE RUB

1 teaspoon onion powder

¾ teaspoon salt

½ teaspoon freshly ground black pepper

½ teaspoon garlic powder

¼ teaspoon cumin

¼ teaspoon paprika

⅛ teaspoon ginger

FOR THE STEAK

1 (1- to 1½-pound) hanger steak

4 tablespoons butter

PER SERVING
RATIO: 4:1
CALORIES: 672
TOTAL FAT: 51.3g
CARBS: 8.9g
NET CARBS: 7.9g
FIBER: 1g
PROTEIN: 43.1g

To make the cilantro crema

1. In a food processor, add the scallions, cilantro, garlic, lime rind, and lime juice. Pulse until the scallions and cilantro emulsify.
2. Add the mayonnaise, sour cream, and salt. Pulse until combined. Refrigerate until ready to serve.

To make the rub

In a small bowl, mix together the onion powder, salt, pepper, garlic powder, cumin, paprika, and ginger.

(continued)

To make the steak

1. Liberally coat the steak with the rub. Set aside.

2. In a large skillet over medium high heat, heat the butter for about 2 minutes, being careful not to burn it.

3. Add the seasoned steak to the skillet. Sear for 3 minutes on each side for rare; 4 minutes per side for medium-rare.

4. Remove the steak from the pan and tent with aluminum foil. Allow the steak to cool for 7 to 10 minutes before slicing.

5. Serve the sliced steak with the cilantro crema on the side.

MEATY MAINS

CHIPOTLE COFFEE-CRUSTED BONE-IN RIB EYE

SERVES 2

PREP TIME: 5 MINUTES ■ COOK TIME: 20 MINUTES ■ TOTAL TIME: 1½ HOURS

Smoky chipotle pairs with the rich, deep flavor of coffee to create a unique steak rub in this rib-eye recipe. A personal favorite often made for birthdays and special occasions, I also like to whip this recipe out when I'm trying to impress someone very special. Best served with simple steamed vegetables like asparagus and broccoli, this steak would also go well with Cauliflower Mac and Cheese (page 96). If I want to make the meal really decadent, I like pairing the steak with Bleu Cheese Sauce (page 217) for additional fat.

FOR THE RUB

1 teaspoon finely ground coffee

¾ teaspoon chipotle powder

½ teaspoon unsweetened cocoa powder

¼ teaspoon onion powder

¼ teaspoon garlic powder

¼ teaspoon salt

¼ teaspoon freshly ground black pepper, finely ground

⅛ teaspoon ground cinnamon

FOR THE STEAK

1 (12- to 14-ounce) bone-in rib-eye steak

2 tablespoons butter

MEATY MAINS

PER SERVING

RATIO: 4:1

CALORIES: 666

TOTAL FAT: 59.9g

CARBS: 1.6g

NET CARBS: 0.9g

FIBER: 0.7g

PROTEIN: 27.5g

To make the rub

In a medium bowl, mix together the coffee, chipotle powder, cocoa powder, onion powder, garlic powder, salt, pepper, and cinnamon.

To make the steak

1. On a parchment-covered cutting board, coat the steak completely with the rub, being sure to get the rub deep into the meat. Wrap the steak in the parchment paper and refrigerate to marinate for at least 1 hour.

2. In a large oven-safe skillet over medium-high heat, melt the butter for 90 seconds.

(continued)

3. Add the steak to the skillet and sear it for 5 to 7 minutes per side for medium-rare. Remove the steak from the skillet. Place it on a plate to rest for at least 5 minutes.

4. Serve the steak with your preferred side dishes.

INGREDIENT TIP: Bone-in rib eye is one of the best beef cuts you can use while on the keto diet due to the high fat content. Even well-marbled steaks can easily lose their tenderness if overcooked, but a bone-in cut gives you more wiggle room when cooking due to the heat having to permeate the bone.

MEATY
MAINS

BEEF BRISKET WITH CAULIFLOWER SALAD

SERVES 14

PREP TIME: 35 MINUTES ▪ COOK TIME: 7 HOURS ▪ TOTAL TIME: 7½ HOURS

Beef brisket can be one of the easiest cuts of meat to cook, but it can also be finicky. Texas barbecue enthusiasts spend years perfecting the right smoking techniques to achieve the perfect flavor. For this recipe, liquid smoke does just fine. Served alongside a keto-friendly "potato salad," this is perfect for a weekend with friends or family. If you do not have a slow cooker, cook the beef brisket in a Dutch oven in a 250°F oven for the same amount of time.

FOR THE CAULIFLOWER SALAD

3½ cups cauliflower florets

4 hardboiled eggs, roughly chopped

1 cup mayonnaise

2 tablespoons mustard

1 teaspoon minced garlic

½ teaspoon salt

¼ teaspoon freshly ground black pepper

¼ teaspoon paprika

1 cup chopped onion

3 tablespoons minced dill pickles

1 teaspoon chopped fresh parsley

FOR THE RUB

2 tablespoons powdered stevia, or other sugar substitute

2 tablespoons paprika

1 tablespoon garlic powder

1 tablespoon onion powder

1 teaspoon cayenne pepper

1 tablespoon ground cumin

1 teaspoon salt

1 tablespoon freshly ground black pepper

1 tablespoon chili powder

FOR THE BRISKET

1 (7- to 8-pound) beef brisket

2 tablespoons olive oil

1½ cups beef stock, divided

1 cup chopped onion

1 tablespoon liquid smoke

PER SERVING

RATIO: 3:1

CALORIES: 749

TOTAL FAT: 52.5g

CARBS: 18g

NET CARBS: 15.9g

FIBER: 2.1g

PROTEIN: 57g

To make the cauliflower salad

1. Bring a large pot of water to a boil. Add the cauliflower and cook for 10 minutes, or until tender. Drain the cauliflower. Set aside in a large bowl to cool.

(continued)

2. Once cooled, roughly chop the cauliflower. Add the eggs and stir to combine.

3. In another large bowl, whisk together the mayonnaise, mustard, garlic, salt, pepper, and paprika. Add the cauliflower and egg mixture, onions, pickles, and parsley. Mix thoroughly to combine. Refrigerate, covered, for at least 2 hours, or until ready to serve.

To make the rub

In a medium bowl, mix together the stevia, paprika, garlic powder, onion powder, cayenne pepper, cumin, salt, black pepper, and chili powder.

MEATY MAINS

To make the brisket

1. Cover the beef brisket with the rub, massaging it into the meat thoroughly.

2. In a large skillet over medium-high heat, heat the olive oil for 1 minute. Add the brisket to the skillet. Brown on all sides for about 3 minutes per side. Once browned, remove the beef brisket from the skillet. Set aside.

3. Add ½ cup of beef stock to the skillet and scrape the bottom of the pan to loosen any browned bits. Remove the skillet from the heat and pour the drippings into a large slow cooker.

4. To the slow cooker, add the remaining 1 cup of beef stock, onions, and liquid smoke. Whisk to combine with the drippings.

5. Add the brisket to the slow cooker. Spoon some liquid over it to coat. Cover and cook on low for 6 hours, 30 minutes, or until tender.

6. Serve the brisket sliced and with a spoonful of the cauliflower salad.

DOUBLE BACON CHEESEBURGER

SERVES 4

PREP TIME: 10 MINUTES ▪ COOK TIME: 20 MINUTES ▪ TOTAL TIME: 30 MINUTES

Is there anything more satisfying than a cheeseburger? I think not. Though this recipe is conspicuously missing the bun, you'll still be impressed by the juicy flavor of the meat combined with the gooey, melted American cheese. Topped with thick-cut bacon, this burger can be eaten alone or served in a lettuce wrap; I personally forgo the lettuce and just dig right in, usually munching on little bites as I plate the rest of the food.

1 pound 80 percent lean ground beef

1 shallot, minced

1 teaspoon minced garlic

1 tablespoon Worcestershire sauce

½ teaspoon salt

¼ teaspoon freshly ground black pepper

4 (1-ounce) slices thick-cut bacon, cooked, grease reserved and cooled

1 tablespoon butter

4 (1-ounce) slices American cheese

4 low-carb buns or lettuce wraps (optional)

PER SERVING
(1 BACON-AND-CHEESE-TOPPED PATTY)

RATIO: 4:1

CALORIES: 585

TOTAL FAT: 42.8g

CARBS: 3.3g

NET CARBS: 3.3g

FIBER: 0g

PROTEIN: 42.5g

1. In a large bowl, mix together the ground beef, shallot, garlic, Worcestershire sauce, salt, pepper, and reserved bacon grease. Divide the mixture into 4 equal portions and form into patties.

2. In a large cast iron (or other heavy-bottomed) skillet over medium-high heat, heat the butter for 1 minute.

3. Add the patties to the skillet and cook for 3 to 4 minutes. Flip and cook 2 to 3 minutes more for medium-rare.

4. Lower the heat to medium-low. Place 1 slice of cheese on each patty. Cover the skillet and melt the cheese for 1 to 2 minutes.

5. Remove the patties from the skillet. Top each with 1 slice of bacon.

6. Serve with your favorite condiments, on a low-carb bun, or with a lettuce wrap (if using).

BEEF FAJITAS

SERVES 3

PREP TIME: 15 MINUTES = COOK TIME: 20 MINUTES = TOTAL TIME: 35 MINUTES

Fajitas are a Mexican favorite and are very keto friendly when you remove the carb-laden tortillas they're usually served with. The serrano pepper adds spice, which can be tempered by omitting it. Pair with low-carb tortillas and sour cream for an authentic flavor.

PER SERVING
(1 FAJITA)
RATIO: 3:1
CALORIES: 749
TOTAL FAT: 52.5g
CARBS: 18g
NET CARBS: 15.9g
FIBER: 2.1g
PROTEIN: 57g

FOR THE RUB

1 teaspoon cumin

½ teaspoon chili powder

½ teaspoon garlic powder

½ teaspoon onion powder

¼ teaspoon paprika

¼ teaspoon salt

¼ teaspoon freshly ground black pepper

FOR THE STEAK

1 (1-pound) skirt steak

3 tablespoons olive oil, divided

1 red bell pepper, sliced

1 green bell pepper, sliced

1 jalapeño pepper, sliced

1 serrano pepper, minced

1 onion, sliced

2 garlic cloves, minced

2 tablespoons fresh cilantro, chopped

1 lime, quartered

3 low-carb tortillas (optional)

To make the rub

In a large bowl, mix together the cumin, chili powder, garlic powder, onion powder, paprika, salt, and pepper.

To make the steak

1. Coat the steak with the rub, massaging it thoroughly into the meat. Set aside.

2. In a large skillet over medium-high heat, heat 1 tablespoon of olive oil for 1 minute. Add the red peppers, green peppers, jalapeño peppers, serrano peppers, onions, and garlic. Sauté for 6 to 7 minutes, until browned and tender. Transfer the pepper and onion mixture to a bowl. Set aside.

3. Add 1 more tablespoon of olive oil to the skillet. Heat on medium-high for 1 minute. Place the seasoned steak into the pan and sear it for 3 to 4 minutes per side for medium-rare. Remove the steak from the skillet. Set aside to rest for at least 3 minutes.

4. Add the remaining tablespoon of olive oil to the skillet. Heat on medium-high heat for 1 minute.

5. Add the peppers and onions back into the skillet. Sauté for 2 minutes.

6. Slice the steak into ¼-inch-thick strips. Add the steak strips to the skillet with the peppers. Cook for 2 to 3 minutes until browned. Add the chopped cilantro. Remove from the heat.

7. Serve garnished with a lime wedge and with the low-carb tortillas (if using) or in Cheesy Taco Shells (page 106).

MEATY MAINS

POT ROAST WITH TURNIPS AND RADISHES

SERVES 6

PREP TIME: 35 MINUTES • COOK TIME: 7 HOURS • TOTAL TIME: 7½ HOURS

Pot roast is a weeknight classic at my house and also serves as a hearty comfort food. While potatoes and carrots aren't allowed on the keto diet, I like to substitute other root vegetables like turnips or radishes for a similar texture and equally great flavor. My tried-and-true secret of thickening the gravy with heavy cream instead of flour also yields a uniquely rich take on this family favorite dish.

1 (4- to 5-pound) bottom round rump roast

¾ teaspoon salt

½ teaspoon freshly ground black pepper

3 tablespoons olive oil

1 onion, quartered

3 cups beef stock, divided

2 garlic cloves

2 fresh thyme sprigs

2 turnips, peeled, roughly chopped

2 cups radishes, halved

¼ cup heavy (whipping) cream

1. Preheat the oven to 475°F.

2. Season the roast with the salt and pepper.

3. In a large Dutch oven over medium-high heat, heat the olive oil for 1 minute. Add the roast to the pot. Brown on all sides, about 3 minutes per side. Once browned, remove it and set aside.

4. Add the onion to the pot and brown for about 3 minutes, stirring. Remove the onion. Set them aside with the roast.

5. Pour ½ cup of beef stock into the pot, scraping the bottom of the pan to loosen any browned bits.

6. Add the remaining 2½ cups of beef stock, the garlic, and thyme to the pot. Whisk to combine.

7. Add the roast and onion back into the pot. Place the turnips and radishes in the pot, surrounding the roast.

8. Place the pot, uncovered, into the preheated oven. Immediately reduce the heat to 400°F and cook for 6 to 6½ hours, or until the internal temperature reaches 130°F. Remove the roast from the oven and allow it to cool for 2 to 3 minutes. Transfer the roast and vegetables to a dish.

9. Into a large saucepan over medium-high heat, pour the remaining liquid from the Dutch oven. Add the heavy cream. Bring the liquid to a boil. Reduce the heat to medium and let the sauce reduce for 4 to 5 minutes.

10. Slice the pot roast and serve with the reduced sauce and vegetables.

COOKING TIP: While the USDA recommends cooking beef to a minimum of 145°F, meat continues to cook after it is removed from the heat. For a juicier, more tender pot roast, allow the meat to cook the additional 10°F while resting. If the meat does not reach 145°F after resting, return it to the heat.

BEEF STROGANOFF

SERVES 4

PREP TIME: 15 MINUTES   COOK TIME: 7 HOURS   TOTAL TIME: 7½ HOURS

Though typically made with noodles, this beef stroganoff recipe uses cabbage to achieve a similar texture with a minimal amount of carbohydrates. Cabbage is also high in nutrients like vitamin C, which keeps your immune system healthy. Store a portion of this dish in the freezer for a quick weeknight meal.

1 (1-pound) beef roast

¼ teaspoon salt

¼ teaspoon freshly ground black pepper

1 tablespoon olive oil

½ cup diced onion

1 cup chopped mushrooms

1 teaspoon minced garlic

4 cups sliced cabbage

1½ cups beef broth

½ cup heavy (whipping) cream

½ cream cheese, at room temperature

1 teaspoon tomato paste

MEATY MAINS

PER SERVING

RATIO: 3:1

CALORIES: 438

TOTAL FAT: 26.9g

CARBS: 8.1g

NET CARBS: 5.8g

FIBER: 2.3g

PROTEIN: 40.4g

1. Season the roast with the salt and pepper. Set aside.

2. In a large skillet over medium-high heat, heat the olive oil for about 1 minute. Add the roast to the skillet Brown on all sides, about 2 minutes per side. Remove the roast from the skillet, reserving any juices, and set aside.

3. Add the onion, mushrooms, and garlic to the skillet. Cook for 2 minutes, or until tender.

4. In a large slow cooker, layer the cabbage on the bottom. Top with the roast. Transfer the onion mixture to the cooker.

5. In a large bowl, mix together the beef broth, heavy cream, cream cheese, and tomato paste. Add to the slower cooker and cover.

6. Cook the roast on low for about 7 hours.

7. With a fork or tongs, shred the roast. Serve with the cabbage.

FIVE-ALARM BEEF CHILI

SERVES 12

PREP TIME: 30 MINUTES · COOK TIME: 2 HOURS · TOTAL TIME: 2½ HOURS

Get ready to turn up the heat with this five-pepper beef chili recipe. Made with bell peppers, poblano peppers, jalapeño peppers, serrano peppers, and some extra-spicy habanero peppers, this chili is great topped with cheese and sour cream. If you prefer a lower level of heat, reduce the amount of habanero peppers to one, or omit them completely.

Don't forget to wear gloves, wash your hands after handling the peppers, and be careful not to touch your face, eyes, or other sensitive skin.

FOR THE CHILI

3 tablespoons olive oil

2 cups diced onion

5 garlic cloves, minced

2 green bell peppers, diced

2 poblano peppers, diced

3 serrano peppers, minced

3 jalapeño peppers, diced

2 to 3 habanero peppers, minced (adjust for heat level; optional)

3 pounds 80 percent lean ground beef

1 cup tomato paste

2¼ cups crushed tomatoes

1½ cups diced tomatoes

2 cups dark beer

1½ tablespoons dark chili powder

½ teaspoon paprika

1 teaspoon salt

1 teaspoon freshly ground black pepper

½ teaspoon cumin

FOR THE TOPPINGS

2 cups shredded Cheddar cheese

1 cup sour cream

Chopped fresh cilantro, for garnish (optional)

MEATY

PER SERVING

RATIO: 3:1

CALORIES: 532

TOTAL FAT: 33.9g

CARBS: 14.9g

NET CARBS: 11g

FIBER: 3.9g

PROTEIN: 38.8g

To make the chili

1. In a large stockpot over medium heat, heat the olive oil for 1 minute. Add the onion and garlic. Cook for 3 minutes until tender.

2. Add the bell peppers, poblano peppers, serrano peppers, jalapeño peppers, and habanero peppers (if using) to the pot. Mix well. Cook for 3 to 4 minutes.

(continued)

3. Add the ground beef to the peppers and onions. Crumble with the back of a spoon while browning for 4 minutes.

4. Add the tomato paste, crushed tomatoes, and diced tomatoes to the pot. Mix well.

5. Add the beer. Increase the heat to high and bring the mixture to a boil.

6. Once the chili boils, cover and lower the heat to medium-low. Cook for 1½ hours.

7. Add the chili powder, paprika, salt, pepper, and cumin. Stir to incorporate. Cook for 5 more minutes, stirring occasionally.

8. Serve the chili with the shredded cheese and sour cream. Garnish with cilantro (if using).

FRUGAL TIP: Buy ground beef in large amounts, like five pounds, then portion into one-pound packages and freeze. Defrost and cook as needed. Many grocers will have a monthly sale on keto staples like ground beef and bacon, so keep an eye out in your weekly paper for the best time to buy.

GROUND BEEF TACO SALAD

SERVES 4

PREP TIME: 30 MINUTES ▪ COOK TIME: 20 MINUTES ▪ TOTAL TIME: 50 MINUTES

Taco salad is one of the easiest recipes to whip up on a busy weeknight. The best part about this recipe is that the taco meat can be doubled and reserved for other dishes, such as the Cheesy Taco Shells (page 106). This recipe freezes well, but be sure to thaw completely before reheating.

FOR THE TACO MEAT

2 tablespoons olive oil

½ cup diced onion

2 garlic cloves, minced

1 green bell pepper, diced

1 jalapeño pepper, diced

6 ounces diced tomatoes, divided

1 pound 80-percent lean ground beef

½ teaspoon cumin

½ teaspoon paprika

¼ teaspoon salt

¼ teaspoon freshly ground black pepper

1 avocado, diced

FOR THE TOPPINGS

½ cup shredded Cheddar cheese

¼ cup sour cream

Fresh cilantro, chopped

PER SERVING

RATIO: 3:1

CALORIES: 587

TOTAL FAT: 44.5g

CARBS: 10.9g

NET CARBS: 5.8g

FIBER: 5.1g

PROTEIN: 36.6g

To make the taco meat

1. In a large skillet over medium-high heat, heat the olive oil for about 1 minute. Add the onion and garlic. Cook for 2 minutes, until tender.

2. Add the bell pepper, jalapeño pepper, and 3 ounces of diced tomatoes to the skillet. Cook for 3 to 4 more minutes.

3. Transfer the mixture to a large bowl. Set aside. Reserve any liquid left in the skillet and place back over the heat.

4. Add the ground beef to the skillet. Cook for 8 to 10 minutes, crumbling the meat, until browned.

5. Add the cumin, paprika, salt, and pepper. Stir to combine.

6. Transfer the beef to the large bowl with the onion and pepper mixture. Toss to combine.

   (continued)

7. Mix in the remaining 3 ounces of tomatoes.

8. Gently stir in the avocado. Do not overmix.

9. Plate each serving of taco salad with a portion of the Cheddar cheese, sour cream, and cilantro toppings.

MEATY
MAINS

PHILLY CHEESESTEAK STUFFED PEPPERS

SERVES 3

PREP TIME: 15 MINUTES · COOK TIME: 25 MINUTES · TOTAL TIME: 40 MINUTES

Without bread, it's hard to imagine a proper Philly Cheesesteak, but you won't miss the original when you cut into one of these stuffed peppers. Rich in all the flavors of the traditional sandwich, this recipe gets an added dose of fat from the mayonnaise used as a binder. If you're still craving the bread, follow the recipe until it comes time to stuff the peppers and instead, place the meat on two slices of Almond Butter Bread (page 104). Put the open-faced sandwich under the broiler for 3 to 4 minutes to brown the meat and cheese.

4 green bell peppers, seeded, tops reserved, plus ¼ cup thinly sliced green bell pepper from reserved tops

3 tablespoons butter

¼ cup chopped onion

1 pound shaved beefsteak

1 garlic clove, minced

1 teaspoon salt

1 teaspoon freshly ground black pepper

½ teaspoon paprika

½ teaspoon ground coriander

¼ teaspoon dill

¼ teaspoon crushed red pepper flakes

½ teaspoon garlic powder

½ teaspoon onion powder

8 slices pepper Jack cheese, divided

2½ tablespoons mayonnaise

PER SERVING
(1 STUFFED PEPPER)

RATIO: 3:1

CALORIES: 585

TOTAL FAT: 42.5g

CARBS: 11.7g

NET CARBS: 8.6g

FIBER: 3.1g

PROTEIN: 38.2g

1. Preheat the oven to 400°F.

2. Slice a thin piece from the bottom of each whole bell pepper so it will not tip over. Place the 4 peppers on a baking sheet and into the preheated oven. Bake for 10 to 15 minutes.

3. In a large skillet over medium-high heat, heat the butter for 1 minute. Add the onions and sliced green bell peppers. Cook for 3 minutes.

4. Add the steak, garlic, salt, black pepper, paprika, coriander, dill, red pepper flakes, garlic powder, and onion powder. Cook for 6 to 7 minutes until the meat browns completely, breaking up the meat as it cooks. Lower the heat to medium-low.

(continued)

5. Remove the whole bell peppers from the oven. Place 1 slice of pepper Jack cheese in each pepper.

6. Transfer the steak mixture to a medium bowl and continue to shred the meat. Add the mayonnaise and mix well to combine.

7. Stuff each pepper with an equal amount of the meat mixture. Top each pepper with 1 of the remaining 4 cheese slices.

8. Place the stuffed peppers back in the oven. Cook for 5 to 7 minutes, or until the cheese melts. Remove from the oven.

9. Serve immediately.

MEATY
MAINS

BANGERS AND CAULIFLOWER MASH

SERVES 4

PREP TIME: 10 MINUTES · COOK TIME: 25 MINUTES · TOTAL TIME: 35 MINUTES

Bangers and mash is a traditional English meal that can become keto-friendly in a snap by substituting Cauliflower Mash (page 99) for the usual mashed potatoes. Use any type of sausage you prefer, but traditional Italian varieties tend to taste best.

8 Italian sausage links

½ teaspoon salt

¼ teaspoon freshly ground black pepper

2 tablespoons olive oil

2 tablespoons butter

1½ cups sliced onions

1 cup beef stock

2 tablespoons sherry (optional)

¼ cup heavy (whipping) cream

Cauliflower Mash (page 99) for serving

MEATY
MAINS

1. In a large skillet over high heat, brown the sausages on all sides, cooking for 5 to 7 minutes. Season with salt and pepper while cooking. Transfer to a plate and set aside.

2. In the same large skillet, over medium-high heat, heat the olive oil and butter for about 1 minute. Add the onions. Cook until they brown, about 7 minutes.

3. Add the beef stock and sherry (if using) to the onions. Stir to combine and bring to a boil. Cook to reduce the liquid, about 4 minutes.

4. Lower the heat to medium. Add the heavy cream to the onion mixture. Cook for another 2 to 3 minutes.

5. Return the sausages and any accumulated juices to the skillet. Cook for 1 minute.

6. Plate two sausages with a serving of Cauliflower Mash per person.

PER SERVING
(2 SAUSAGE LINKS, PLUS CAULIFLOWER MASH)

RATIO: 4:1

CALORIES: 583

TOTAL FAT: 52.3g

CARBS: 10.5g

NET CARBS: 7.6g

FIBER: 2.9g

PROTEIN: 17.8g

ZUCCHINI MEATLOAF

SERVES 7

PREP TIME: 20 MINUTES   COOK TIME: 1 HOUR   TOTAL TIME: 1½ HOURS

Meatloaf is a staple food that many people grew up with, but that was a different breed of meatloaf entirely. Although meatloaf is usually bulked up with oats or bread crumbs, this recipe relies on zucchini and added fat from bacon to achieve the same texture. Serve a slice of this meatloaf with some Cauliflower Mash (page 99) for a hearty and heartwarming meal.

1 pound 80-percent lean ground beef

½ pound bacon, chopped

1 zucchini, finely chopped

1 onion, finely chopped

3 tablespoons tomato paste

2 eggs

1 tablespoon Dijon mustard

¼ teaspoon paprika

¼ teaspoon salt

¼ teaspoon freshly ground black pepper

1¼ cups almond flour

Cooking spray for loaf pan

PER SERVING
RATIO: 3:1
CALORIES: 517
TOTAL FAT: 36.9g
CARBS: 8g
NET CARBS: 4.8g
FIBER: 3.2g
PROTEIN: 32g

1. Preheat the oven to 350°F.

2. In a large bowl, combine the ground beef, bacon, zucchini, and onion.

3. Add the tomato paste, eggs, mustard, paprika, salt, and pepper. Mix thoroughly to combine.

4. Add the almond flour and mix again, making sure there are no clumps.

5. Transfer the beef mixture to a loaf pan coated with cooking spray. Cover with aluminum foil and place in the preheated oven. Cook for 1 hour.

6. Take the loaf from the oven and remove the foil. Return the loaf to the oven.

7. Increase the heat to broil. Cook for 10 minutes, or until the top is browned.

8. Remove the pan from the oven. Allow the meatloaf to cool in the pan for 5 minutes.

9. Run a knife along the inside edges of the pan to remove the meatloaf.

10. Slice into 7 equal slices and serve.

BAKED CHEESY MEATBALLS

SERVES 3

PREP TIME: 20 MINUTES • COOK TIME: 40 MINUTES • TOTAL TIME: 1 HOUR

Traditional Italian meatballs are a beauty to behold. Their texture is hard to replicate without the use of bread crumbs, but a mixture of almond flour and Parmesan cheese stands in quite nicely. Combined with sugar-free Pasta Sauce (page 224) and heaps of mozzarella cheese, this dish pairs perfectly with a plate of Zucchini Noodles (page 121) or is just as delicious on its own.

½ pound 80-percent lean ground beef

½ pound ground pork

½ cup grated Parmesan cheese

¼ cup almond flour

2 tablespoons water

1 tablespoon minced garlic

½ teaspoon salt

¼ teaspoon freshly ground black pepper

1 tablespoon olive oil

2 tablespoons butter

1½ cups Pasta Sauce (page 224), or purchased sugar-free marinara

¾ cup shredded mozzarella cheese

Fresh parsley for garnish

1. Preheat the oven to 400°F.

2. In a large bowl, combine the ground beef, pork, Parmesan cheese, almond flour, water, garlic, salt, and pepper. Mix thoroughly. Form the meat into about 10 small meatballs.

3. In a large skillet over medium-high heat, heat the olive oil and butter for about 1 minute.

4. Add the meatballs to the skillet. Brown on all sides, about 2 minutes per side. Remove from the skillet. Set aside.

5. In an oven-safe dish, arrange the meatballs to fill the dish with no large empty space.

6. Cover the meatballs with the Pasta Sauce. Top the meatballs evenly with the mozzarella.

7. Place the dish into the preheated oven. Bake for 15 to 20 minutes, until the cheese browns and the internal temperature of the meatballs is 170°F.

8. Garnish with the parsley, and serve.

MEATY MAINS

PER SERVING
(ABOUT 3
MEATBALLS)

RATIO: 3:1

CALORIES: 672

TOTAL FAT: 39.8g

CARBS: 9.7g

NET CARBS: 7.6g

FIBER: 2.1g

PROTEIN: 62.1g

BEEF AND BROCCOLI STIR-FRY

SERVES 4

PREP TIME: 30 MINUTES • COOK TIME: 20 MINUTES • TOTAL TIME: 50 MINUTES

Straight from your favorite Chinese takeout kitchen, this beef and broccoli dish eliminates hidden carbs like cornstarch and sugar for a tasty meal. Try this with Cauliflower "Rice" (page 98) or tossed with Zucchini Noodles (page 121).

2 tablespoons soy sauce

2 garlic cloves, minced

2 tablespoons sake

1 tablespoon grated fresh ginger

½ teaspoon Chinese five-spice powder

1 (1-pound) skirt steak, sliced into 1-inch strips, then halved crosswise

3 tablespoons coconut oil

1 cup diced onion

4 cups broccoli florets

½ cup sliced scallions

MEATY MAINS

PER SERVING
RATIO: 3:1
CALORIES: 378
TOTAL FAT: 22g
CARBS: 11.8g
NET CARBS: 7.3g
FIBER: 3.5g
PROTEIN: 33.9g

1. In a large bowl, mix together the soy sauce, garlic, sake, ginger, and five-spice powder. Add the steak strips. Cover. Refrigerate to marinate for at least 15 minutes.

2. In a large deep skillet or wok over medium-high heat, heat the coconut oil for about 1 minute. Add the onion. Sauté for 2 minutes, or until tender.

3. Add the beef and marinade to the skillet. Cook for 4 to 5 minutes, stirring occasionally.

4. Add the broccoli and scallions to the skillet. Sauté for 2 minutes. Cover and reduce the heat to medium-low. Cook, covered, for another 2 to 3 minutes, or until the broccoli is tender.

5. Stir the ingredients to mix well, and serve.

SERVING TIP: Plate this with a scoop of Cauliflower "Rice" (page 98) for a Chinese takeout experience you'll swear is the real deal. For extra toasted or fried rice, use 1 teaspoon of oil per 1 cup of Cauliflower "Rice" and toast over medium-high heat for 3 minutes before serving.

HERB-CRUSTED LAMB CHOPS

SERVES 3

PREP TIME: 15 MINUTES   COOK TIME: 15 MINUTES   TOTAL TIME: 30 MINUTES

Fresh herbs play off the rich flavor of lamb in this herb-crusted recipe. Best served with simple side dishes like Cauliflower Mash (page 99) and steamed vegetables, this classic preparation is the perfect way to impress your guests with minimal effort. Do not substitute dried herbs for fresh in this recipe, as the bright flavor of the fresh herbs is what makes this simple dish so delicious.

1 pound lamb chops

2 tablespoons Dijon mustard

4 fresh rosemary sprigs, chopped

4 fresh thyme sprigs, chopped

3 tablespoons almond flour

4 garlic cloves, minced

1 teaspoon onion powder

¼ teaspoon salt

¼ teaspoon freshly ground black pepper

4 tablespoons olive oil, divided

PER SERVING

RATIO: 3:1

CALORIES: 486

TOTAL FAT: 32.1g

CARBS: 3.9g

NET CARBS: 2.6g

FIBER: 1.3g

PROTEIN: 43.3g

1. Preheat the oven to 350°F.

2. Coat the lamb chops with the mustard. Set aside.

3. To a blender or food processor, add the rosemary, thyme, almond flour, garlic, onion powder, salt, and pepper. Pulse until finely chopped. Slowly add about 2 tablespoons of olive oil to form a thick paste.

4. Press the herb paste firmly around the edges of the mustard-coated chops, creating a crust.

5. In a large oven-safe skillet over medium heat, heat the remaining 2 tablespoons of olive oil for 2 minutes. Add the chops to the skillet on their sides to brown. Cook, undisturbed, for 2 to 3 minutes so the crust adheres properly to the meat. Turn and cook on the opposite edge for 2 to 3 minutes more. Transfer the chops to a baking sheet.

6. Place the sheet in the preheated oven. Cook for 7 to 8 minutes, for medium.

7. Remove the sheet from the oven. Serve immediately.

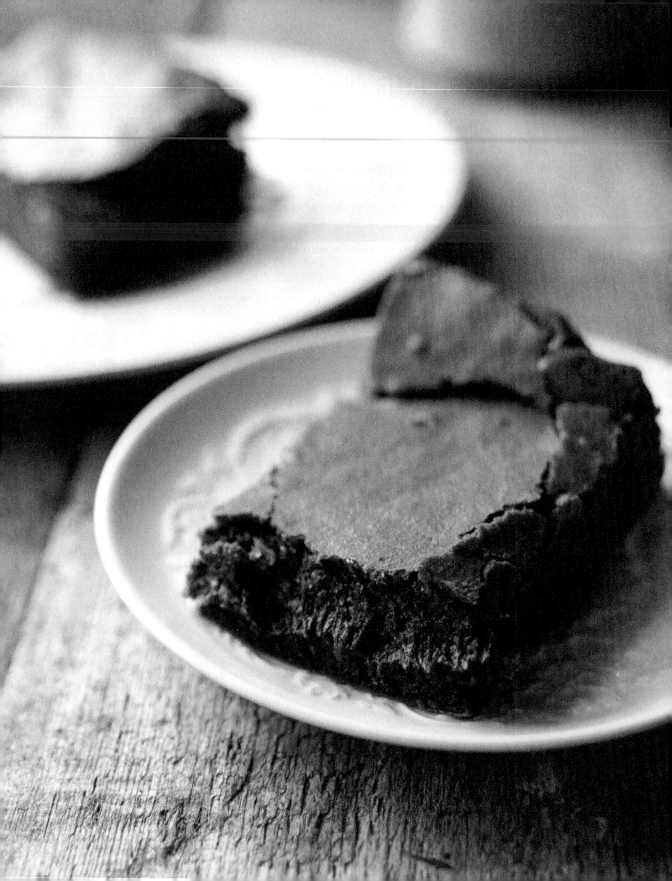

CHAPTER

9

DELIGHTFUL DESSERTS

COCONUT LEMON FAT BOMBS

SERVES 16

TOTAL TIME: 1¼ HOURS

Fat bombs are the perfect dessert to help you reach your fat macronutrient goal for the day. These Coconut Lemon Fat Bombs get a punch from lemon extract to help the lemon flavor shine through. Add unsweetened coconut flakes for added texture.

2 ounces cream cheese

4 tablespoons butter

4 tablespoons coconut oil

4 tablespoons heavy (whipping) cream

2 tablespoons freshly squeezed lemon juice

1 teaspoon lemon extract

1 teaspoon stevia, or other sugar substitute

PER SERVING
(1 BOMB)

RATIO: 4:1

CALORIES: 81

TOTAL FAT: 8.9g

CARBS: 0.4g

NET CARBS: 0.4g

FIBER: 0.4g

PROTEIN: 0.4g

1. To a medium microwaveable bowl, add the cream cheese, butter, and coconut oil. Microwave on high in short 10-second intervals until the mixture begins to melt. Once melted, add the heavy cream. Whisk thoroughly to combine.

2. Mix in the lemon juice, lemon extract, and stevia.

3. Pour the mixture evenly into an ice cube tray. Freeze for at least 1 hour to solidify, preferably overnight.

4. Enjoy within 2 hours.

INGREDIENT TIP: If lemon extract and lemon juice are not lemony enough for you, grate some lemon rind and add 1 teaspoon to the mixture. Meyer lemons have an intense flavor, so use them when possible.

CHOCOLATE PEANUT BUTTER FAT BOMBS

SERVES 16

TOTAL TIME: 1¼ HOURS

When my legendary chocolate cravings hit, I reach for these peanut buttery cups of high-fat bliss. This recipe seamlessly blends coconut oil with peanut butter powder to create a smooth texture. If I only have regular peanut butter on hand, I just decrease the amount of coconut oil by about 1 tablespoon. My favorite way to eat these is to take small bites and let them slowly melt. De-li-cious.

4 tablespoons butter

4 tablespoons coconut oil

4 tablespoons heavy (whipping) cream

2 tablespoons powdered peanut butter, like PB2

2 tablespoons unsweetened cocoa powder

1 teaspoon pure vanilla extract

1 teaspoon stevia, or other sugar substitute

1. To a medium microwaveable bowl, add the butter and coconut oil. Microwave on high in short 10-second intervals until the mixture begins to melt. Once melted, add the heavy cream. Whisk thoroughly to combine.

2. Mix in the powdered peanut butter, cocoa powder, vanilla, and stevia.

3. Pour the mixture evenly into an ice cube tray. Freeze for at least 1 hour to solidify, preferably overnight.

4. Enjoy within 2 hours.

DELIGHTFUL DESSERTS

PER SERVING (1 BOMB)

RATIO: 4:1

CALORIES: 73

TOTAL FAT: 7.8g

CARBS: 1g

NET CARBS: 0.5g

FIBER: 0.5g

PROTEIN: 0.6g

BLUEBERRY CREAM CHEESE BITES

SERVES 16

TOTAL TIME: 1 ¼ HOURS

Almost like cheesecake, these Blueberry Cream Cheese Bites are quite the treat. Sweetened naturally by the berries, this minimal-ingredient recipe is perfect to keep in the freezer for a sweet snack. Try these with blackberries or raspberries, as well.

4 tablespoons butter

¼ cup cream cheese

4 tablespoons coconut oil

4 tablespoons heavy (whipping) cream

¼ cup blueberries, finely chopped

1 teaspoon pure vanilla extract

DELIGHTFUL DESSERTS

PER SERVING
(1 BITE)
RATIO: 4:1
CALORIES: 82
TOTAL FAT: 8.9g
CARBS: 0.6g
NET CARBS: 0.6g
FIBER: 0g
PROTEIN: 0.4g

1. To a medium microwaveable bowl, add the butter, cream cheese, and coconut oil. Microwave on high in short 10-second intervals until the mixture begins to melt. Once melted, add the heavy cream and blueberries.

2. Transfer the mixture to a blender. Pulse to blend in the blueberries.

3. Add the vanilla and pulse to combine.

4. Pour the mixture evenly into an ice cube tray. Freeze for at least 1 hour to solidify, preferably overnight.

5. Treat yourself within 2 hours.

MINIATURE CHEESECAKES

SERVES 12

PREP TIME: 10 MINUTES ▪ COOK TIME: 35 MINUTES ▪ TOTAL TIME: 50 MINUTES

In my opinion, cheesecake is the almost-perfect keto dessert—except for its sugar and crust. Here, I make the crust with almond flour and the filling with stevia instead of cane sugar. When one of those chocolate cravings hits, I like to add chunks of dark chocolate or small pieces of fruit. Play around with your favorite add-ins to the make this dessert recipe your own.

4 tablespoons butter

½ cup almond flour

2 cups cream cheese, at room temperature

¾ cup stevia, or other sugar substitute

1 teaspoon pure vanilla extract

½ teaspoon freshly squeezed lemon juice

DELIGHTFUL DESSERTS

1. Preheat the oven to 300°F.
2. In a medium microwaveable bowl, microwave the butter on high for 20 seconds, or until melted. Add the almond flour to the bowl. Mix to combine.
3. In a cupcake pan, divide the almond flour crust evenly among the cups. Press the mixture firmly into the bottom of each. Place the pan in the preheated oven. Bake for 10 minutes. Remove from the oven. Set aside.
4. In a large bowl, mix together the cream cheese, stevia, vanilla, and lemon juice.
5. Top each crust with an equal amount of the cream cheese batter.
6. Return the pan to the oven. Bake for 15 minutes.
7. Increase the heat to 350°F. Bake for 10 minutes more.
8. Remove from the oven. Cool for 5 minutes.

PER SERVING
(1 MINI CHEESECAKE)

RATIO: 3:1

CALORIES: 227

TOTAL FAT: 19.5g

CARBS: 13.9g

NET CARBS: 13.4g

FIBER: 0.5g

PROTEIN: 2.9g

LEMON CHEESECAKE BARS

SERVES 8

PREP TIME: 10 MINUTES ▪ COOK TIME: 2 HOURS ▪ TOTAL TIME: 2½ HOURS

An almond flour base is accented with a creamy lemon topping in this recipe. The sugar-free gelatin and almond flour crust are what make this recipe keto-friendly. If you have it on hand, dust these bars with powdered stevia for added garnish.

½ cup butter, melted

½ cup almond flour

1 cup boiling water

⅓ cup sugar-free lemon gelatin mix

8 ounces (1 package) cream cheese

2 tablespoons freshly squeezed lemon juice

PER SERVING
(1 LEMON BAR)
RATIO: 4:1
CALORIES: 268
TOTAL FAT: 25.2g
CARBS: 2.1g
NET CARBS: 1.3g
FIBER: 0.8g
PROTEIN: 6.5g

1. Preheat the oven to 350°F.

2. In a medium bowl, mix together the melted butter and the almond flour. Transfer the mixture to an 8-inch-square baking pan. Press the mixture firmly into the bottom to form a crust.

3. Place the pan in the preheated oven. Bake for 10 minutes. Remove from the oven. Set aside to cool.

4. In large bowl, combine the boiling water and gelatin. Stir for about 2 minutes to dissolve.

5. Add the cream cheese and lemon juice. Mix well to combine.

6. Pour the cream cheese mixture over the cooled crust. Refrigerate for at least 2 hours until set, preferably overnight.

7. Cut into 8 bars and serve.

COCONUT TRUFFLES

SERVES 12

TOTAL TIME: 25 MINUTES

Unsweetened coconut flakes wrap around rich cream cheese for these quick and easy truffles. Extremely simple, these can be frozen and thawed as needed or refrigerated in an airtight container. Experiment by adding spices, like cinnamon, for a twist.

8 ounces (1 package) cream cheese, at room temperature

½ cup stevia, or other sugar substitute

2 teaspoons coconut extract

½ cup unsweetened shredded coconut

1. In a medium bowl, mix together the cream cheese, stevia, and coconut extract.

2. Scoop into balls, 1 to 2 tablespoons in size. It should yield about 12.

3. Roll the balls in the coconut flakes. Chill the truffles for 15 minutes before serving.

DELIGHTFUL
DESSERTS

PER SERVING
(1 TRUFFLE)
RATIO: 4:1
CALORIES: 98
TOTAL FAT: 9.3g
CARBS: 1.6g
NET CARBS: 0.9g
FIBER: 0.7g
PROTEIN: 1.8g

CHOCOLATE MUG CAKE

SERVES 1

TOTAL TIME: 10 MINUTES

This is the keto-version of the now-famous chocolate mug cake. Made with stevia instead of sugar and aided by extra egg, this fluffy, delicious chocolate cake will delight you. Top with whipped cream or serve with fresh berries for an added treat.

Cooking spray

2 tablespoons cocoa powder

2 tablespoons stevia, or other sugar substitute

Pinch salt

1 tablespoon heavy (whipping) cream

½ teaspoon pure vanilla extract

1 egg, beaten

¼ teaspoon baking powder

PER SERVING
(1 CAKE)
RATIO: 3:1
CALORIES: 146
TOTAL FAT: 11.3g
CARBS: 7.5g
NET CARBS: 4.3g
FIBER: 3.2
PROTEIN: 7.8g

1. Spray the inside of a microwaveable mug with cooking spray.

2. In a medium bowl, mix together the cocoa powder, stevia, and salt.

3. Add the heavy cream, vanilla, and the beaten egg. Mix to combine. Add the baking powder and mix again.

4. Continue mixing until there are no air bubbles.

5. Transfer the batter to the prepared mug. Microwave on high for 1 minute, 20 seconds.

6. Remove the cake from the microwave. Allow it to settle for 1 minute before inverting onto a plate to serve.

DOUBLE CHOCOLATE BROWNIES

SERVES 8

PREP TIME: 10 MINUTES ▪ COOK TIME: 30 MINUTES ▪ TOTAL TIME: 45 MINUTES

Rich, dark chocolate is the shining star in this double chocolate brownie recipe. Sprinkled with dark chocolate, these gooey, almond flour–based brownies are good to the last crumb. Garnish with a dollop of whipped cream or some sliced berries.

¾ cup almond flour

½ cup stevia, or other sugar substitute

3 tablespoons cocoa powder

½ teaspoon baking powder

¼ teaspoon salt

4 tablespoons butter, melted

3 eggs

1 teaspoon pure vanilla extract

¼ cup 90 percent dark chocolate, crumbled

1. Preheat the oven to 350°F.
2. In a large bowl, combine the almond flour, stevia, cocoa powder, baking powder, and salt. Whisk to combine.
3. In a medium bowl, whisk together the butter, eggs, and vanilla.
4. Add the butter mixture to the almond flour. Stir to combine.
5. Incorporate the dark chocolate into the batter. Transfer the batter to an 8-inch-square baking pan.
6. Place the pan in the preheated oven. Cook for 30 minutes.
7. Remove the pan from the oven. Cool the brownies for at least 5 minutes before cutting into 8 portions.

PER SERVING
(1 BROWNIE)

RATIO: 4:1

CALORIES: 191

TOTAL FAT: 17.2g

CARBS: 5.5g

NET CARBS: 2.9g

FIBER: 2.6g

PROTEIN: 3.2g

PEANUT BUTTER COOKIES

MAKES 25

PREP TIME: 10 MINUTES · COOK TIME: 13 MINUTES · TOTAL TIME: 25 MINUTES

Peanut butter and cream cheese come together to create this unique, chewy cookie. Crunchy on the outside but chewy on the inside, these mimic the traditional peanut butter cookie in many ways. The dough will be very sticky, so wet your hands before forming the cookies.

1 cup sugar-free peanut butter

½ cup cream cheese, at room temperature

20 drops liquid stevia, or other liquid sugar substitute

1 egg

1 teaspoon pure vanilla extract

PER SERVING
(1 COOKIE)
RATIO: 3:1
CALORIES: 79
TOTAL FAT: 6.9g
CARBS: 2.2g
NET CARBS: 1.6g
FIBER: 0.6 g
PROTEIN: 3.1g

1. Preheat the oven to 350°F.

2. In a large bowl, combine the peanut butter, cream cheese, stevia, egg, and vanilla. Mix thoroughly to combine. Divide the dough by heaping tablespoons into 25 equal portions. Form into balls.

3. On parchment-lined baking sheets, arrange the cookie balls at least 1 inch apart.

4. With a fork, flatten each cookie, crisscrossing the imprint with the tines.

5. Place the baking sheets in the oven. Bake for 12 to 13 minutes, or until golden brown.

6. Cool the cookies for 2 to 3 minutes before serving. Store in an airtight container.

CHOCOLATE-COVERED BACON

SERVES 4

PREP TIME: 15 MINUTES ▪ COOK TIME: 20 MINUTES ▪ TOTAL TIME: 1½ HOURS

Chocolate and bacon, two of life's most sinful pleasures, come together in this decadent, savory, and sweet recipe. Skewering the bacon allows the chocolate to adhere well to the meat, though it is not necessary. If you work without the skewers, simply cook the bacon flat in a pan, transfer to parchment paper, and brush on the chocolate.

8 bacon slices

1½ tablespoons coconut oil

3 tablespoons unsweetened chocolate chips or pieces

1 teaspoon stevia, or other sugar substitute

1. Preheat the oven to 425°F.

2. Skewer each bacon slice accordion-style.

3. Place on a baking sheet. Put the sheet in the preheated oven. Bake for 15 minutes, until crisp.

4. Remove the bacon from the oven and cool completely.

5. In a medium saucepan over low heat, melt the coconut oil and chocolate. Whisk in the stevia.

6. Transfer the bacon to a sheet of parchment paper. With a pastry brush, coat one side of each bacon slice with some of the chocolate. Flip. Coat the other side of each piece with the remaining chocolate.

7. Refrigerate for 1 hour before serving.

PER SERVING
(2 CHOCOLATE-COVERED BACON SLICES)

RATIO: 3:1

CALORIES: 214

TOTAL FAT: 12.8g

CARBS: 3.2g

NET CARBS: 1.8g

FIBER: 1.4g

PROTEIN: 9.4g

ZUCCHINI MUFFINS

SERVES 16

PREP TIME: 5 MINUTES · COOK TIME: 20 MINUTES · TOTAL TIME: 30 MINUTES

These light, easy-to-make zucchini muffins are handy to have for a quick breakfast. They are excellent paired with Cinnamon Butter (page 227) and a cup of Buttered Coffee (page 32). Refrigerate in an airtight container to preserve the quality.

1 cup grated, drained zucchini

1 cup almond flour

¾ cup almond butter

3 eggs

1 tablespoon honey

1 teaspoon pure vanilla extract

1 teaspoon baking powder

1 teaspoon cinnamon

PER SERVING
(1 MUFFIN)
RATIO: 3:1
CALORIES: 184
TOTAL FAT: 14.9g
CARBS: 6.7g
NET CARBS: 4.9g
FIBER: 1.8g
PROTEIN: 4.8g

1. Preheat the oven to 350°F.

2. In a large bowl, combine the zucchini, almond flour, almond butter, eggs, honey, vanilla, baking powder, and cinnamon. Mix well.

3. Line a cupcake pan with paper liners. Divide the batter evenly among the paper liners.

4. Place the pan in the preheated oven. Bake for 18 to 20 minutes, or until golden brown.

5. Cool the muffins for 5 minutes before serving.

CHOCOLATE COCONUT MILK ICE CREAM

SERVES 1

TOTAL TIME: 35 MINUTES

Ice cream is not very keto-friendly, but when made this unique way with coconut milk you get the same creamy consistency without the added sugar. Enjoy this with unsweetened coconut flakes, cocoa nibs, or shaved dark chocolate. You can make vanilla-flavored ice cream by replacing the cocoa powder with 1 teaspoon of vanilla extract.

½ cup coconut milk

1 tablespoon heavy (whipping) cream

1 tablespoon unsweetened cocoa powder

1. In a large bowl, whisk the coconut milk, heavy cream, and cocoa powder for 2 minutes, until it thickens and forms stiff peaks.
2. Transfer the mixture to a freezer-safe container. Freeze for 20 to 30 minutes, until set to your desired consistency.

PER SERVING
(1 RECIPE)

RATIO: 4:1

CALORIES: 340

TOTAL FAT: 34.9g

CARBS: 10g

NET CARBS: 5.6g

FIBER: 4.4g

PROTEIN: 4.1g

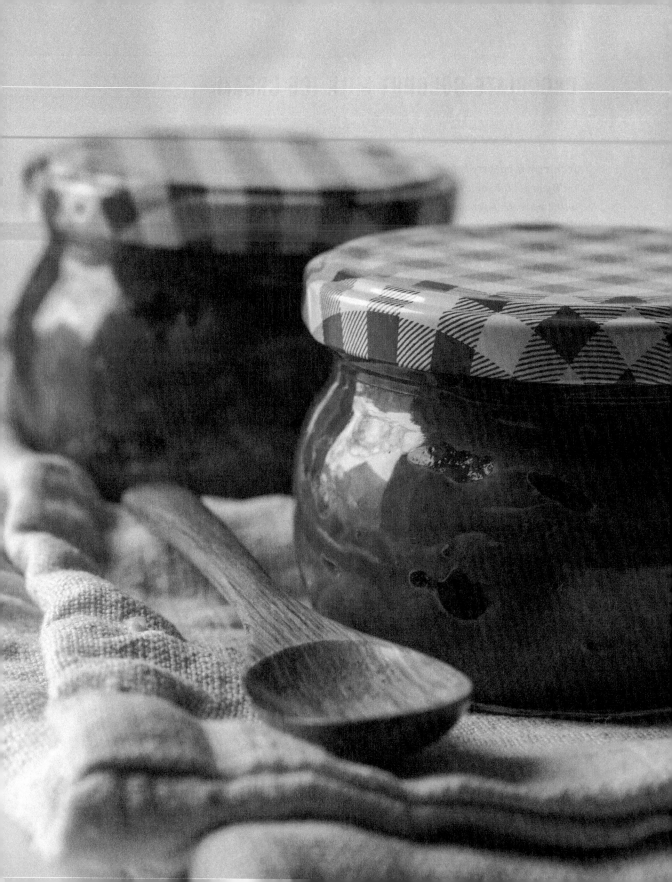

CHAPTER

10

KITCHEN STAPLES: CONDIMENTS, SAUCES, & DRESSINGS

BARBECUE SAUCE

YIELDS 10 SERVINGS

PREP TIME: 10 MINUTES • COOK TIME: 30 MINUTES • TOTAL TIME: 40 MINUTES

Almost all barbecue sauces are laden with sugar, which was a real deal breaker for me as a Texan on the keto diet. Undeterred by the lackluster flavor of most bottled sugar-free barbecue sauces, which can also be very expensive, I randomly chose to whip up a batch of this sauce and lo-and-behold, it tasted almost as good as the stuff you'll get at the finest barbecue joints. It goes well on almost everything: baked chicken, pork ribs, pulled pork . . . the list goes on. Enjoy this sauce right after making it, then store in an airtight container in the refrigerator for up to two weeks.

PER SERVING
(1 TABLESPOON)
RATIO: 3:1
CALORIES: 47
TOTAL FAT: 2.2g
CARBS: 6.6g
NET CARBS: 5.2g
FIBER: 1.4g
PROTEIN: 1.7g

1 tablespoon butter

½ cup finely chopped onion

1½ tablespoons minced garlic

1¼ cups sugar-free cola

¾ cup tomato paste

½ cup water

¼ cup Sugar-Free Ketchup (page 216)

1 tablespoon Worcestershire sauce

3 tablespoons mustard

1 teaspoon cayenne pepper

1 teaspoon liquid smoke

½ teaspoon paprika

½ teaspoon freshly ground black pepper

1. In a large saucepan over medium-high heat, heat the butter for about 1 minute. Add the onion. Cook until translucent, about 4 minutes. Add the garlic and cook for 1 minute.

2. Add the cola, tomato paste, water, Sugar-Free Ketchup, Worcestershire sauce, mustard, cayenne, liquid smoke, paprika, and pepper. Whisk well to combine.

3. Bring the sauce to a simmer. Cook for 25 minutes, stirring occasionally, until thickened.

TERIYAKI SAUCE

YIELDS 8 SERVINGS
PREP TIME: 10 MINUTES   COOK TIME: 15 MINUTES   TOTAL TIME: 25 MINUTES

Much like barbecue sauce, teriyaki sauce is also a hiding place for sugar. Use this recipe if you're out of store-bought teriyaki, or tinker with it to suit your personal tastes. Teriyaki sauce will store in an airtight container for about 2 weeks.

⅓ cup olive oil

1 teaspoon minced garlic

1 tablespoon minced fresh ginger

1 cup tamari soy sauce

2 tablespoons Worcestershire sauce

2 tablespoons white vinegar

20 drops liquid stevia, or other liquid sugar substitute

½ teaspoon freshly ground black pepper

¼ teaspoon orange extract

1. In a large saucepan over medium-high heat, heat the olive oil for about 1 minute. Add the garlic and ginger. Cook for 1 minute, until fragrant.

2. Add the tamari, Worcestershire sauce, vinegar, stevia, pepper, and orange extract. Whisk to combine. Bring to a boil. Reduce to a simmer and cook for 15 minutes, until reduced by about half.

3. Store in an airtight container or use immediately.

KITCHEN STAPLES

PER SERVING
(1 TABLESPOON)

RATIO: 3:1

CALORIES: 110

TOTAL FAT: 8.4g

CARBS: 3.5g

NET CARBS: 3.4g

FIBER: 0.1g

PROTEIN: 4.1g

SUGAR-FREE KETCHUP

YIELDS 16 SERVINGS
TOTAL TIME: 1¼ HOURS

Ketchup always surprises dieters with how sugary it can be. While the natural sugars in tomatoes are usually enough to get the right flavor, most packaged ketchups also contain added sugar. To make your own sugar-free keto-ketchup, try this simple recipe.

1½ cups tomato paste

¼ cup water

4 tablespoons apple cider vinegar

2 tablespoons Worcestershire sauce

1 tablespoon mustard

½ teaspoon salt

½ teaspoon cinnamon

¼ teaspoon garlic powder

⅛ teaspoon freshly ground black pepper

⅛ teaspoon ground cloves

1. In a large bowl, combine the tomato paste, water, cider vinegar, Worcestershire sauce, mustard, salt, cinnamon, garlic powder, pepper, and cloves. Whisk thoroughly to combine.

2. Transfer to an airtight container. Chill for 1 hour to allow the flavors to incorporate.

KITCHEN STAPLES

PER SERVING
(1 TABLESPOON)
RATIO: 3:1
CALORIES: 24
TOTAL FAT: 0.3g
CARBS: 4.8g
NET CARBS: 3.8
FIBER: 1g
PROTEIN: 1.1g

BLEU CHEESE SAUCE

YIELDS 8 SERVINGS
PREP TIME: 10 MINUTES · COOK TIME: 1 HOUR · TOTAL TIME: 1¼ HOURS

Thick, creamy, and perfect for dipping vegetables and buffalo chicken wings, bleu cheese is one of the most flavorful sauces out there. Usually thickened with flour, this recipe uses almond flour to create the base before mixing with a large amount of bleu cheese.

1 tablespoon butter

1 tablespoon almond flour

½ cup chicken broth

½ cup heavy (whipping) cream

¼ cup unsweetened almond milk

4 ounces bleu cheese

1. In a large saucepan over medium-high heat, melt the butter. Add the almond flour and reduce the heat to low. Cook for 2 to 3 minutes, whisking constantly.

2. Add the chicken broth, heavy cream, and almond milk. Whisk to combine. Increase the heat to medium.

3. Add the bleu cheese. Whisk to combine until the cheese melts and the sauce is creamy in texture.

4. Pour the sauce into a bowl and place in the refrigerator to chill for at least 1 hour.

5. Refrigerate in an airtight container for up to 1 week.

KITCHEN STAPLES

PER SERVING
(1 TABLESPOON)
RATIO: 3:1
CALORIES: 98
TOTAL FAT: 8.9g
CARBS: 0.7g
NET CARBS: 0.6g
FIBER: 0.1g
PROTEIN: 3.5g

RANCH DRESSING

YIELDS 16 SERVINGS

PREP TIME: 10 MINUTES — COOK TIME: 1 HOUR — TOTAL TIME: 1¼ HOURS

While not always the case, many ranch dressings contain hidden carbs. To avoid packing on 10 grams of carbs while binging on vegetables and ranch dressing, use this recipe instead.

1 cup mayonnaise

1 cup sour cream

¼ cup buttermilk

1 tablespoon onion powder

1 tablespoon dried parsley

2 teaspoons garlic powder

½ teaspoon salt

½ teaspoon dried dill

½ teaspoon mustard powder

¼ teaspoon celery salt

PER SERVING
(1 TABLESPOON)
RATIO: 3:1
CALORIES: 93
TOTAL FAT: 8g
CARBS: 5g
NET CARBS: 4.8g
FIBER: 0.2g
PROTEIN: 0.9g

1. In a large bowl, mix together the mayonnaise, sour cream, buttermilk, onion powder, parsley, garlic powder, salt, dill, mustard powder, and celery salt. Whisk well to incorporate.

2. Refrigerate for 1 hour before serving.

3. Refrigerate in an airtight container for up to 2 weeks.

ALFREDO SAUCE

YIELDS 6 SERVINGS
PREP TIME: 5 MINUTES ▪ COOK TIME: 10 MINUTES ▪ TOTAL TIME: 15 MINUTES

This basic white sauce is perfect for chicken, zucchini noodles, or served with a grilled steak. Almond flour thickens the sauce in lieu of flour, and almond milk tempers the thickness of heavy cream to smooth out the texture.

2 tablespoons butter

2 tablespoons almond flour

⅛ teaspoon freshly ground black pepper

¼ teaspoon salt

⅛ teaspoon paprika

½ cup unsweetened almond milk

½ cup heavy (whipping) cream

3 tablespoons sour cream

1. In a large saucepan over low heat, melt the butter. Add the almond flour, pepper, salt, and paprika. Whisk until smooth.
2. Slowly add the almond milk, stirring constantly to avoid forming lumps.
3. Add the heavy cream and sour cream. Continue to whisk.
4. Cook on low for 8 to 10 minutes, or until thickened.
5. Refrigerate in an airtight container for up to 1 week.

KITCHEN STAPLES

PER SERVING
(1 TABLESPOON)
RATIO: 3:1
CALORIES: 99
TOTAL FAT: 10.3g
CARBS: 1g
NET CARBS: 1g
FIBER: 0g
PROTEIN: 0.5g

MUSTARD CREAM SAUCE

YIELDS 6 SERVINGS

PREP TIME: 5 MINUTES · COOK TIME: 10 MINUTES · TOTAL TIME: 15 MINUTES

This sour cream–based, mustard-flavored sauce complements grilled meats and baked chicken. Use spicy mustard for more of a bite, or add 1 teaspoon of apple cider vinegar for a thinner consistency.

1 tablespoon butter

1 tablespoon minced onion

1 teaspoon minced garlic

½ cup heavy (whipping) cream

½ cup sour cream

1 tablespoon mustard

¼ teaspoon salt

⅛ teaspoon freshly ground black pepper

KITCHEN STAPLES

1. In a large saucepan over low heat, melt the butter. Add the onion and garlic. Cook for 5 minutes, until tender.
2. Add the heavy cream and sour cream. Whisk until the consistency begins to thin.
3. Whisk in the mustard, salt, and pepper. Remove from the heat.
4. Allow the sauce to cool. Refrigerate in an airtight container for up to 1 week.

PER SERVING
(1 TABLESPOON)
RATIO: 3:1
CALORIES: 103
TOTAL FAT: 10.2g
CARBS: 2.1g
NET CARBS: 1.9g
FIBER: 0.2g
PROTEIN: 1.4g

HOMEMADE MAYONNAISE

YIELDS 32 SERVINGS
TOTAL TIME: 15 MINUTES

Homemade mayonnaise is a real treat if you have time to make it. Prepackaged condiments have made our lives easier, but nothing beats the taste of fresh mayonnaise.

2 teaspoons mustard powder

2 tablespoons freshly squeezed lemon juice, divided

1 teaspoon salt

1 teaspoon stevia, or other sugar substitute

⅛ teaspoon freshly ground black pepper

2 egg yolks, preferably pasteurized

1¾ cups canola oil, divided

2 tablespoons vinegar

1. Fill a large bowl with ice. Nestle a medium bowl into the ice.

2. To the medium bowl, add the mustard powder, 1 tablespoon of lemon juice, salt, stevia, and pepper. With an electric mixer, beat thoroughly.

3. Add the egg yolks, mixing well on medium-high speed.

4. Very slowly, while continuing to mix, add ¼ cup of canola oil, teaspoon by teaspoon. Slowly continue to add the remaining 1½ cups of oil while mixing steadily.

5. When the mixture begins to thicken, continue mixing and add the vinegar and the remaining tablespoon of lemon juice intermittently with the oil. Continue until all ingredients are added and all the oil has been used.

6. Refrigerate in an airtight container for up to 1 week. Do not freeze.

KITCHEN STAPLES

PER SERVING
(1 TABLESPOON)
RATIO: 4:1
CALORIES: 110
TOTAL FAT: 12.3g
CARBS: 0.1g
NET CARBS: 0.1g
FIBER: 0g
PROTEIN: 0.2g

HOLLANDAISE SAUCE

YIELDS 8 SERVINGS
TOTAL TIME: 10 MINUTES

Hollandaise is the perfect sauce to top your breakfast eggs with, and it is great to have on hand while on the keto diet. This easy preparation for hollandaise will save you the expense of going out to a pricey brunch to experience this decadent sauce.

2 egg yolks, preferably pasteurized

¼ teaspoon salt

½ cup butter, melted

1 tablespoon lemon juice

1. To a large bowl, add the egg yolks and beat with an electric mixer until they are thick and lemon-colored. Add the salt.

2. While continuing to beat constantly, slowly add the butter, 1 teaspoon at a time, alternating with the lemon juice, ½ teaspoon at a time. Beat constantly until the sauce is smooth.

3. Refrigerate in an airtight container for up to 3 days.

KITCHEN STAPLES

PER SERVING
(1 TABLESPOON)
RATIO: 4:1
CALORIES: 116
TOTAL FAT: 12.7g
CARBS: 0.2g
NET CARBS: 0.2g
FIBER: 0g
PROTEIN: 0.8g

MUSTARD SHALLOT VINAIGRETTE

YIELDS 8 SERVINGS
TOTAL TIME: 10 MINUTES

Faced with the need to eat more salads, I knew whatever I put on my greens needed to burst with flavor. Tangy mustard pairs with the bite of shallot in this bright vinaigrette. Perfect for salads or as a marinade, this dressing is incredibly versatile and will quickly become a staple in your kitchen, like it has in mine.

½ cup olive oil

½ cup apple cider vinegar

3 tablespoons Dijon mustard

1 shallot, minced

½ teaspoon salt

¼ teaspoon freshly ground black pepper

1. In a blender or food processor, add the olive oil, cider vinegar, mustard, shallot, salt, and pepper.
2. Pulse for about 1 minute, until combined.
3. Refrigerate in an airtight container for up to 2 weeks.

KITCHEN STAPLES

PER SERVING
(1 TABLESPOON)
RATIO: 4:1
CALORIES: 117
TOTAL FAT: 12.8g
CARBS: 0.9g
NET CARBS: 0.9g
FIBER: 0g
PROTEIN: 0.3g

PASTA SAUCE

YIELDS 8 SERVINGS

PREP TIME: 5 MINUTES · COOK TIME: 10 MINUTES · TOTAL TIME: 15 MINUTES

Many canned tomato and pasta sauces are chock-full of sugars. Skip the carbs in prepackaged pasta sauces by making this sugar-free recipe.

3 cups diced tomatoes

¼ cup olive oil

2 tablespoons minced garlic

1 tablespoon chopped fresh basil

1 teaspoon onion powder

1 teaspoon crushed red pepper flakes

½ teaspoon salt

¼ teaspoon freshly ground black pepper

1. In a blender or food processor, add the tomatoes and pulse once or twice so the tomatoes still have texture.

2. In a large saucepan over medium heat, heat the olive oil for about 1 minute. Add the garlic. Cook for 1 minute, until fragrant.

3. Add the tomatoes, basil, onion powder, red pepper flakes, salt, and pepper to the saucepan.

4. Whisk to combine. Bring the mixture to a simmer. Cook for 10 minutes. Remove from the heat and allow to cool.

5. Refrigerate in an airtight container for up to 3 weeks. Freezes well.

KITCHEN STAPLES

PER SERVING
(1 TABLESPOON)

RATIO: 3:1

CALORIES: 69

TOTAL FAT: 6.5g

CARBS: 3.3g

NET CARBS: 2.5g

FIBER: 0.8g

PROTEIN: 0.7g

PIZZA SAUCE

YIELDS 16 SERVINGS
TOTAL TIME: 15 MINUTES

Thicker than pasta sauce and slightly more flavorful, this pizza sauce recipe is perfect on the Cauliflower Pizza (page 101) or Cheesy-Crust Pizza (page 103). Add fresh herbs like parsley and thyme for a more pronounced herb flavor.

2 cups diced tomatoes

¼ cup olive oil

¼ cup chopped onion

2 tablespoons minced garlic

1 cup tomato paste

2 teaspoons onion powder

1 teaspoon crushed red pepper flakes

½ teaspoon salt

¼ teaspoon freshly ground black pepper

3 tablespoons chopped fresh basil

1. In a blender or food processor, add the tomatoes and pulse once or twice so the tomatoes still have texture.

2. In a large saucepan over medium heat, heat the olive oil for about 1 minute. Add the onion and garlic. Cook for 2 minutes, until tender.

3. Add the tomatoes, tomato paste, onion powder, red pepper flakes, salt, and pepper to the saucepan. Stir to combine. Bring to a simmer. Cook for 10 minutes. Remove from the heat and allow to cool.

4. Add the basil. Stir to incorporate.

5. Refrigerate in an airtight container for up to 3 weeks.

KITCHEN STAPLES

PER SERVING
(1 TABLESPOON)
RATIO: 3:1
CALORIES: 46
CARBS: 4.3g
TOTAL FAT: 3.3g
NET CARBS: 3.4g
FIBER: 0.9g
PROTEIN: 0.9g

PESTO SAUCE

YIELDS 14 SERVINGS
TOTAL TIME: 15 MINUTES

Fresh basil, pine nuts, and Italian cheeses blend together to create a kitchen staple that is loved for its intense fresh flavor. Pesto is a delicate sauce. Treat it gently so as not to bruise the basil unnecessarily.

4 cups fresh basil, chopped

½ cup olive oil

⅓ cup pine nuts

2 garlic cloves, minced

¼ cup freshly grated Parmesan cheese

¼ cup freshly grated pecorino cheese

1 teaspoon salt

1. In a blender or food processor, add the basil, olive oil, pine nuts, and garlic. Pulse in short bursts while slowly adding the Parmesan and pecorino cheeses.

2. Add the salt. Blend until smooth.

3. Refrigerate in an airtight container for up to 3 days.

KITCHEN STAPLES

PER SERVING
(1 TABLESPOON)
RATIO: 4:1
CALORIES: 106
TOTAL FAT: 10.9g
CARBS: 0.9g
NET CARBS: 0.7g
FIBER: 0.2g
PROTEIN: 2.6g

CINNAMON BUTTER

YIELDS 16 SERVINGS
TOTAL TIME: 1 HOUR, 15 MINUTES

Compound butter—butter paired with supplementary ingredients—is a way of life. Once you've had it, you'll wonder why you haven't been using it every day. Cinnamon butter pairs well with almost any baked good, and is great between pancakes and on top of waffles. Its uses are endless.

1 cup butter, at room temperature

10 drops liquid stevia, or other liquid sugar substitute

1 teaspoon pure vanilla extract

1 teaspoon ground cinnamon

¼ teaspoon salt

1. In a medium bowl, mix together the butter, stevia, vanilla, cinnamon, and salt. Use a mixer to combine.

2. Spoon the butter onto a sheet of waxed parchment paper, or regular wax paper. Roll into a long log in the center of the paper, leaving about 2 inches of paper on each side of the butter. Roll the paper around the butter and twist the ends.

3. Chill the butter for at least 1 one hour before using. Refrigerate for up to 2 weeks.

KITCHEN STAPLES

PER SERVING
(1 TABLESPOON)

RATIO: 4:1

CALORIES: 103

TOTAL FAT: 11.5g

CARBS: 0.1g

NET CARBS: 0.1g

FIBER: 0g

PROTEIN: 0.1g

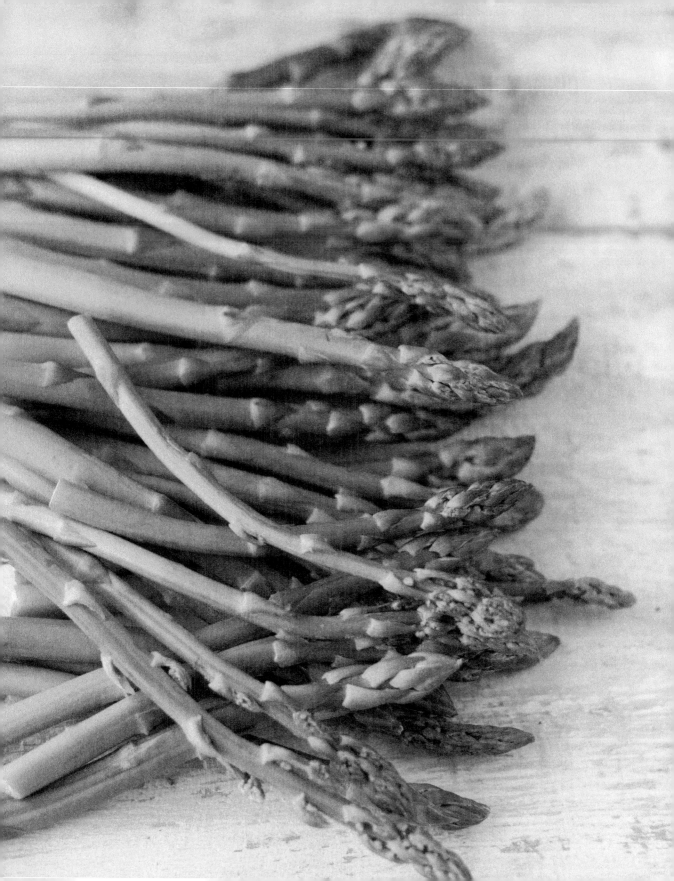

THE DIRTY DOZEN & THE CLEAN FIFTEEN

A nonprofit and environmental watchdog organization called Environmental Working Group (EWG) looks at data supplied by the US Department of Agriculture (USDA) and the Food and Drug Administration (FDA) about pesticide residues and compiles a list each year of the best and worst pesticide loads found in commercial crops. You can use these lists to decide which fruits and vegetables to buy organic to minimize your exposure to pesticides and which produce is considered safe enough to skip the organics. This does not mean they are pesticide-free, though, so wash these fruits and vegetables thoroughly.

These lists change every year, so make sure you look up the most recent before you fill your shopping cart. You'll find the most recent lists as well as a guide to pesticides in produce at EWG.org/FoodNews.

2014 DIRTY DOZEN

Apples	Peaches	*In addition to the dirty dozen, the EWG added two produce contaminated with highly toxic organo-phosphate insecticides:*
Celery	Potatoes	
Cherry tomatoes	Snap peas (imported)	
Cucumbers	Spinach	
Grapes	Strawberries	Blueberries (domestic)
Nectarines (imported)	Sweet bell peppers	Hot peppers

2014 CLEAN FIFTEEN

Asparagus	Eggplants	Papayas
Avocados	Grapefruits	Pineapples
Cabbage	Kiwis	Sweet corn
Cantaloupes (domestic)	Mangoes	Sweet peas (frozen)
Cauliflower	Onions	Sweet potatoes

cacao: Seeds from the cacao tree used to make cocoa and chocolate.

capsaicin: Extract from hot peppers, like jalapeños and habaneros, that causes a burning sensation.

carbohydrate: One of the three major macronutrients serving as the primary energy source for the brain, primarily derived from sugars and starches that digest into glucose. Carbohydrates yield 4 kilocalories per gram.

epilepsy: A neurological disorder that disrupts normal brain activity, causing seizures.

fat: One of the three major macronutrients providing energy to the body. Composed of solid or semisolid triglycerides, fat is found naturally in meat, poultry, fish, and some plant seeds. Fats yield 9 kilocalories per gram.

glucose: A simple sugar that is the primary source of energy for plants and animals.

gluconeogenesis: A metabolic process in which protein is turned into glucose. Excessive protein consumption can stifle the ability to enter a state of ketosis.

glycemic index: Measures the rate at which consumed carbohydrates increase blood glucose levels. Values range from 1 (slowest increase) to 100 (fastest).

insulin: Hormone produced by the pancreas that helps control blood sugar levels, and allows the body to utilize sugar from carbohydrates for energy.

ketoacidosis: A dangerous metabolic state brought on by a lack of insulin in the body and the presence of massive quantities of ketones. Usually seen in type 1 diabetics, this condition should be monitored closely.

ketogenic: Defined by the formation of ketones.

ketone body: Used by the body for energy instead of glucose, ketone bodies are produced by the liver from fatty acids during fasting or while on carb-restricting diets.

ketosis: A metabolic state, achieved through dietary deprivation of sugar, in which the body uses fats as its primary energy. To achieve a state of ketosis, one's net carbohydrate intake must be at or below 20 grams daily.

Ketostix: A brand of testing strips used to measure the level of ketones in the urine.

kilocalorie: Calorie.

low-carb diet: A diet that consists of no more than 50 to 100 grams of net carbohydrate per day.

macronutrient: Carbohydrates, proteins, and fats are the three major macronutrients. They constitute the bulk of our diet, and supply energy and many essential nutrients.

MCT oil: An easily digestible and concentrated form of coconut oil composed of medium chain triglycerides. Processed in the liver, medium chain triglycerides act similarly to carbohydrates, providing energy.

net carbohydrate: Determined by subtracting the amount of fiber consumed daily from the total daily carbohydrate amount. This number is important for understanding overall daily carbohydrate consumption.

protein: One of the three major macronutrients that serves as the major structural component of cells in the body. Protein is found in meat, poultry, seafood, beans, peas, eggs, processed soy products, nuts, and seeds. Each protein yields 4 kilocalories per gram.

ratio: On a ketogenic diet, the ratio (usually 4:1, and sometimes 3:1) indicates that a recipe's dietary units of fat are four, or three, times that of the combined proteins and carbohydrates. This measurement originally comes from the classic ketogenic diet, which was developed for those with seizure disorders and other medical issues.

spiralizer: Kitchen tool that cuts firm vegetables like zucchini into noodle-like shapes, which can then be used in recipes to replace pasta in an effort to control carbohydrate consumption.

stevia: A natural sweetener and sugar substitute derived from the stevia plant. Contains 0 calories, 0 carbs, and has a 0 value on the glycemic index.

sugar alcohol: A class of reduced-calorie sweeteners with a lower glycemic impact than regular sugar. Common examples include xylitol, erythritol, and maltitol.

type 1 diabetes: A disease characterized by the insufficient production of insulin to properly handle glucose in the body. Too much glucose can result in serious complications.

APPENDIX C
CONVERSION TABLES

Volume Equivalents (Liquid)

US STANDARD	US STANDARD (OUNCES)	METRIC (APPROXIMATE)
2 tablespoons	1 fl. oz.	30 mL
¼ cup	2 fl. oz.	60 mL
½ cup	4 fl. oz.	120 mL
1 cup	8 fl. oz.	240 mL
1½ cups	12 fl. oz.	355 mL
2 cups or 1 pint	16 fl. oz.	475 mL
4 cups or 1 quart	32 fl. oz.	1 L
1 gallon	128 fl. oz.	4 L

Oven Temperatures

FAHRENHEIT (F)	CELSIUS (C) (APPROXIMATE)
250	120
300	150
325	165
350	180
375	190
400	200
425	220
450	230

Volume Equivalents (Dry)

US STANDARD	METRIC (APPROXIMATE)
⅛ teaspoon	0.5 mL
¼ teaspoon	1 mL
½ teaspoon	2 mL
¾ teaspoon	4 mL
1 teaspoon	5 mL
1 tablespoon	15 mL
¼ cup	59 mL
⅓ cup	79 mL
½ cup	118 mL
⅔ cup	156 mL
¾ cup	177 mL
1 cup	235 mL
2 cups or 1 pint	475 mL
3 cups	700 mL
4 cups or 1 quart	1 L
½ gallon	2 L
1 gallon	4 L

Weight Equivalents

US STANDARD	METRIC (APPROXIMATE)
½ ounce	15 g
1 ounce	30 g
2 ounces	60 g
4 ounces	115 g
8 ounces	225 g
12 ounces	340 g
16 ounces or 1 pound	455 g

REFERENCES

Brinkworth, G. D., et al. "Long-Term Effects of a Very-Low-Carbohydrate Weight Loss Diet Compared With an Isocaloric Low-Fat Diet after 12 Months." *The American Journal of Clinical Nutrition* 90, no. 1 (July 2009): 23–32.

Dyson, P. A., et al. "A Low-Carbohydrate Diet Is More Effective in Reducing Body Weight Than Healthy Eating in Both Diabetic and Non-Diabetic Subjects." *Diabetic Medicine* 24, no. 12 (December 2007): 1430–5.

Epilepsy Foundation. "Treating Seizures and Epilepsy: Dietary Therapies: Ketogenic Diet." Accessed August 28, 2014. www.epilepsy.com/learn/ treating-seizures-and-epilepsy/ dietary-therapies/ketogenic-diet.

Hession, M., et al. "Systematic Review of Randomized Controlled Trials of Low-Carbohydrate vs. Low-Fat/Low-Calorie Diets in the Management of Obesity and Its Comorbidities." *Obesity Reviews* 10 (January 2009): 36–50. doi: 10.1111/j.1467-789X.2008.00518.x

Paoli, A., A, Rubini, J. S. Volek, and K. A. Grimald. "Beyond Weight Loss: A Review of Therapeutic Uses of Very-Low-Carbohydrate (Ketogenic) Diets." *European Journal of Clinical Nutrition* 67, no.8 (August 2013): 3. doi:10.1038/ ejcn.2013.116.

Samaha, F. F., et al. "A Low-Carbohydrate as Compared with a Low-Fat Diet in Severe Obesity." *New England Journal of Medicine* 348, no. 21 (May 2003): 2074–81.

Volek, J. S., et al. "Comparison of Energy-Restricted Very Low Carbohydrate and Low-Fat Diets on Weight Loss and Body Composition in Overweight Men and Women." *Nutrition and Metabolism* 1 (November 2004): 13. doi:10.1186/1743-7075-1-13.

Yancy, W. S. Jr., et al. "A Low-Carbohydrate, Ketogenic Diet Versus a Low-Fat Diet to Treat Obesity and Hyperlipidemia: A Randomized, Controlled Trial." *Annals of Internal Medicine* 140, no. 10 (May 2004): 769–77.

RESOURCES

Books

Coleman, Ella. *Keto Living Cookbook: Lose Weight with 101 Delicious and Low Carb Ketogenic Recipes.* New York: Visual Magic Productions, 2013.

Davis, William, MD. *Wheat Belly: Lose the Wheat, Lose the Weight, and Find Your Path Back to Health.* New York: Rodale Books, 2011.

McDonald, Lyle. *The Ketogenic Diet.* New York: Morris Publishing, 1998.

Moore, Jimmy. *Keto Clarity: Your Definitive Guide to the Benefits of a Low-Carb, High-Fat Diet.* New York: Victory Belt Publishing, 2014.

Taubes, Gary. *Good Calories, Bad Calories: Fats, Calories, and the Controversial Science of Diet and Health.* New York: Anchor, 2008.

——. *Why We Get Fat: And What to Do About It.* New York: Knopf, 2010.

Volek, Jeff S., PhD, RD, and Stephen D. Phinney, MD, PhD. *The Art and Science of Low Carbohydrate Performance.* New York: Beyond Obesity LLC, 2012.

Websites

For further information about the keto diet, visit the following:

CavemanKeto.com

Examine.com

AllRecipes.com/recipes/healthy-recipes/special-diets/low-carb/

LowCarbDiets.about.com

Bodybuilding.com

CharlieFoundation.org

DietDoctor.com

Epilepsy.com

IBreatheImHungry.com

Keto-Calculator.ankerl.com

MyFitnessPal.com

Netrition.com

Ruled.me

RECIPE INDEX

INDEX